Diverticulitis Cookbook

Healing Recipes for 1500 Days of Relief.
60-Day Meal Plan to Deal with Diverticulitis Flare-Ups Included.

John Davis

Table of Content

Chapter 5: LOW RESIDUE DIET RECIPES

5.1 BREAKFAST

Chapter 6: HIGH FIBER RECIPES 65

6.1 BREAKFAST 65

Introduction

Diverticula are tiny, bulging pouches that may occur in the digestive system's lining. The inflammation or irritation of the pouches that may occur is known as diverticulitis. The pouches are normally harmless. They might appear in the intestines at any time. Diverticulosis is the medical term for having these pouches. Diverticulitis occurs when they get infected or inflamed. They're most often discovered in the big intestine's lower section (colon). Diverticula are frequent beyond the age of 40, and they rarely cause difficulties.

Diverticulosis is the occurrence of diverticula. Diverticulitis may result in severe stomach discomfort, a temperature, nausea, and a significant change in bowel patterns.

The following are some of the signs of diverticulitis:

- Pain is the most common symptom, soreness, or sensitivity in the abdomen's left bottom side. Pain might start mild and gradually worsen over time, or it can strike quickly.
- Fever
- Vomiting or nausea are common side effects.
- Chills
- Lower-abdominal cramping
- Less common is diarrhea or constipation
- There is rectal bleeding

If one does not have any symptoms, they don't require treatment for diverticulosis. Nevertheless, since diverticulosis may progress to diverticulitis, a high-fiber diet is recommended as a preventative approach. Consume more vegetables, fruits, grains, seeds, beans, legumes & nuts while consuming less red meat. Relaxation, dietary adjustments, and antibiotics may all help with mild diverticulitis. Diverticulitis that is severe or recurrent may need surgery.

Chapter 1: Diverticulitis Causes and Symptoms

The digestive disorders diverticular disease & diverticulitis both impact the large intestine. Diverticula are the small pouches or bulges or pouches that may form in the lining of your intestine, especially in older adults. Many patients with diverticula are not aware of their condition & only know of its existence when they go for another treatment. Diverticulosis is a condition in which there are no symptoms.

The following are some of the signs and symptoms of diverticular disease:

Belly discomfort that comes and goes, commonly in the lower left side, and feels worse during or immediately after eating (bowel movement eases it)

- Diarrhea, constipation, or both

- Sometimes, blood might be seen in your feces.

When your diverticula become inflamed and irritated/infected, you may experience the following symptoms:

- Experience more acute belly ache regularly

- A very hot temperature

- If you have mucus or blood in the feces

One possible cause of the disease , which is highly controversial, is the protrusion of such sacs outward from the colon. The main factor, however, is a nutritional deficiency, namely, lack of dietary fiber. Fiber relaxes stools, and not getting enough of it causes hard stools. As muscles force the feces down, this may put greater pressure or stress on the colon. Diverticula are considered to form because of this stress.

Diverticula form when weak places in the colon muscle's outer layer give way, allowing the inner layer to press through. Even though there is no conclusive clinical evidence linking dietary fiber to diverticulosis, experts believe the circumstantial evidence is compelling. However, the subject is a contentious one. Diverticula disease is rare in places with high dietary fiber consumption, such as in Africa or South Asia. In Western nations, on the other hand, where dietary fiber consumption is substantially lower, it is quite common.

Nuts, corn & seeds eating were formerly considered to be a cause of diverticula formation.

Although there is no one known cause of diverticular illness, several factors might raise your chances of getting it, including:

- Genetics
- Immune system dysfunction
- Obesity
- Diet
- A lack of physical activity
- Smoking
- Alterations in the microbiota of the gut
- Steroid medicines
- Diets heavy in red meat and poor in fiber

According to research, some genes will intensify the risk of developing diverticular illness in certain individuals.

Scientists are investigating other elements that may have a role in diverticular illness.

These elements include:

- Germs or feces being trapped in a pocket in the colon
- Alterations in the intestinal microbiome
- In your colon, you may have issues with connective nerves, tissue or muscles.
- Immune system complications

1.3 Taking care of Diverticulitis

It's normally not a reason for alarm if you've been informed you have diverticulosis. This is a prevalent ailment that becomes worse as you get older. It affects nearly half of all persons over the age of 59 and practically everyone over the age of 79. If you have diverticulosis, you will most likely have no symptoms. If your diverticulosis is minor, it may go away without therapy.

Diverticulitis affects up to 30% of patients with diverticulosis. Between 5-15% of people will have colon bleeding.

Most persons with diverticulitis will heal after taking antibiotics for seven to ten days and resting. Rupture of the colon (1-2% of patients), blockage (unusual), fistula (14%), and abscess are the most common severe complications of diverticulitis (30 %).

Eating a high-fiber diet (that is rich in vegetables, cereals, whole grains, fruits, nuts, legumes, and beans) is the best self-treatment. Additionally, increase your hydration intake (half the body weight in oz. per day) and workout (helps speed waste through the colon).

Chapter 2: Diverticulitis Diet Basics

If you have significant diverticulitis symptoms, the doctor may suggest a liquid diverticulitis diet as part of the therapy that may include:

- Fruit juices

- Broth

- Water

- Ice pops

You may gradually return to a normal diet. Before introducing high-fiber meals, the doctor may urge you to begin with clean liquids, then low-fiber foods (meat, poultry, white bread, eggs, dairy products & eggs).

Fiber softens and bulks up feces, traveling through the colon more readily. It also helps to relieve pressure in the intestines. According to research, diverticular symptoms may be controlled by consuming fiber-rich meals. Women under the age of 51 should consume 25 g of fiber each day. Men under the age of 51 should consume 38 g of fiber each day. Women over the age of 51 should consume 21 g of calcium each day. Men over the age of 51 should consume 30 g of protein each day.

While high-fiber meals should be included in your diet, you should limit them if you have a diverticulitis flare-up. You're probably suffering a flare if you're exhibiting symptoms like stomach pain, nausea, vomiting, diarrhea, fever or constipation, and chills. Schedule an appointment with your doctor, who will probably prescribe medication and a clear liquid diet.

A liquid-containing diet is quite limited and is intended to relax your digestive system. Ice chips, fruit juices with no pulp, clear ice pops, gelatin, Water, tea, and coffee are all good options (without milk or cream).

When the signs of the flare have subsided, speak with your doctor to determine whether you're ready to resume eating low-fiber foods. Rice, begin with cooked or canned fruits (without the skins), cooked or canned soft vegetables (without the skins), eggs, low-fiber cereals, fish, milk, rice, yogurt, cheese, pasta & white bread.

You should not attempt to follow this diet without consulting your doctor first. You should resume consuming high-fiber foods after the inflammation has subsided and the doctor has cleared you. Also, be sure you drink enough water.

2.1 Foods to Avoid

Foods to stay away from if you have diverticulitis

- People who follow this diet limit food that are rich in FODMAPS. This comprises, for example, the following foods:
- Thick-skinned unpeeled fruits
- Full-fat dairy products
- Sauerkraut and kimchi are examples of fermented products.
- Meals with a lot of trans fats
- Meats that have been red and cured

According to a study, eating a diet strong in processed & red meat may raise your chance of having diverticulitis. A diet rich in fruits, whole grains, and vegetables may help lower the risk of heart disease.

The typical Western diet is heavy in fat, sugar, and carbohydrate but low in fiber. As a result, a person's chance of having diverticulitis may rise.

According to research, eating the following foods may help prevent or lessen the symptoms of diverticulitis:

- Food that has been fried
- Refined grains
- Red meat

2.2 Foods to eat

For diverticulitis, a clear liquid diet is recommended.

A clear liquid diet may be recommended if a flare-up is serious or necessitates surgery. You graduate from fluids to a low-residue diet in 1-2 days. "Even if your discomfort does not go away, you continue to eat usual foods." You can't stay on a liquid diet for an extended period of time since you'll get malnourished.

Depending upon your flare-up, you can consume the following foods on a clear liquid diet:

- Clear broths

- Juices that are clear and without pulp

- Jell-O.

- Ice pops.

For diverticulitis, a low-fiber diet is recommended. Eat a low-residue or GI gentle diet for milder forms of diverticulitis. Based on the intensity of the flare-up, a low-fiber diet restricts fiber consumption to 8-12 g per day.

Low-fiber foods to consider include:

Grains: White spaghetti and white bread. These, as well as white crackers & white rice, are low-fiber alternatives.

Get the peeler ready for low-fiber starches. Potatoes with no skin are an option. They may be mashed, roasted, or baked. Puffed rice cereal & corn flakes are two low-fiber cereals that receive a nod of approval.

Eggs, seafood, egg whites, meat & tofu are all good protein sources. Chopped-up chicken, light ground beef, and tender baked fish are the finest choices.

Fruits: Be cautious while eating fruits since they contain a lot of fiber. Canned fruits like peaches, pears, ripe bananas, soft, ripe cantaloupe, applesauce, honeydew are all good choices. You're not consuming the skin, so there's not a lot of fiber. Insoluble fiber, which may aggravate inflamed polyps, is found in the skin. If you're recuperating from a flare-up, cottage cheese and Greek yogurt are big winners in fact they're rich in calcium, minerals, & protein, plus they don't have any fiber. They're also soft, creamy, and easier to swallow if you're sick. Milk and cheese are additional options.

2.3 List of things to buy

- Bread, cereals, pasta made with whole grains
- Legumes & beans (chickpeas, kidney beans, lentils, pinto beans)
- Seasonal Fruits
- Berries
- Vegetables (peas, squash & spinach)
- Potatoes, sweet potatoes

- Bulgur
- Whole wheat crackers
- Tortillas
- Green peas
- Broccoli
- Collard greens
- Oatmeal
- Rice, both brown & wild

Chapter 3: 3 Step Diverticulitis Diet

3.1 Stage 1: Clear Liquid Diet

It's critical to assist your digestive system in cleaning itself out and beginning to recover during a flare-up or at the onset of symptoms. Use the clear broths as a starting point.

Consuming bone broths prepared from cattle, chicken, fish, lamb may aid with irritable bowel syndrome, joint mobility, immune system boosting, and even cellulite reduction, all while healing the digestive system.

Bone broths with tender vegetables and a little amount of meat give your body critical elements such as calcium, Sulphur, magnesium & phosphorus and others in an easily digestible form.

You may add veggies to the clear broth, then strain later.

Cook the bone broth for a long time to extract all the flavors & gelatin from them. Gelatin has incredible healing powers, and it may even help people with food allergies and sensitivities handle certain foods better. It also helps to maintain a healthy probiotic balance by breaking down proteins to make them simpler to digest. Probiotics aid in the creation of a healthy digestive environment.

In addition, drink 2-3 cups of warm ginger tea each day to help decrease irritation and assist digestion. Ginger is a nutrient-dense spice that boosts the digestive and immune systems.

Only clear broths, calming teas & clear no-pulp juice should be consumed during the initial phase of the diverticulitis diet.

3.2 Stage Two: Low Fiber, Low Residue Diet

After the symptoms of diverticulitis have subsided, you may go to phase two of the diet, which includes introducing readily digested meals such as grated, cooked, and then blended fruits and veggies while continuing to consume calming teas and broth soups.

Fresh fruits and veggies may be juiced for a nutritional boost. Apples, carrots, grapes, apples, lettuce, watercress & beets may be juiced and consumed throughout this stage. Foods with firm skins and tiny seeds should be avoided since they might clog the diverticula sacs.

These foods are low in fiber

- White bread with no seeds & nuts
- White rice
- Peeled & Cooked vegetables with no seeds
- Dairy products

- Oranges
- Watermelon
- Eggs
- Cantaloupe
- Poultry

3.3 Stage Three: High Fiber Diet

Start adding fiber-rich foods, including fruits and veggies, and unprocessed grains, such as quinoa, fermented grains, lentils & black rice after your body has acclimated to the foods in Phase 2. Although experts assumed that eating seeds and nuts was dangerous, they now feel that it is harmless and may even prevent diverticulitis.

Attend to the body; if you start to suffer symptoms of diverticulitis again, go back to the earlier stage. It might take a few months for your digestive system to fully recover.

Diverticulosis: (signs that are no longer active)

Diverticulitis: (signs that are present)

Symptoms aren't apparent currently, but it's still vital to consume a high-fiber diet to avoid inflammation and constipation.

Fiber-rich foods include:

- Whole wheat bread & pasta
- Broccoli
- Brown rice
- Cauliflower
- Leafy Greens

- Potatoes
- Brussel sprouts
- Whole grains
- Cabbage

Chapter 4: CLEAR LIQUID DIET RECIPES

4.1 BREAKFAST

1. Apple Juice

(Prep time: 10 minutes / Servings: 1)

Ingredients

- 1 apple, peeled & cut into wedges
- Water, as needed

Instructions

- In a blender, add water & apple.
- Blend well until smooth
- Strain over cheesecloth & a strainer. Serve.

Nutrition: Kcal 27 | Protein 0.1 g | Fiber 1.6 g | Carbs 6.7 g | Fat 0.2 g

2. Smooth Sweet Tea

(Prep time: 10 minutes | Cook time: 15 minutes | Servings: 8)

Ingredients

- 6 cups of cool water
- ¾ cup of white sugar
- 2 cups of boiling water
- 6 tea bags

Instructions

- In a pitcher, add tea bags & boiling water. Mix & let it steep for 15 minutes.
- Take the tea bags out & mix with sugar. Add cool water & keep it in the fridge.
- Serve chilled.

Nutrition: Kcal 72 | Protein 0.1 g | Fiber 1.2 g | Carbs 18.7 g | Fat 0.2 g

3. Warm Honey Green Tea

(Prep time: 10 minutes | Cook time: 15 minutes | Servings: 4)

Ingredients

- 4 lemon's peel, cut into strips
- 4 lemon slices
- 4 orange's peel, cut into strips
- 4 cups of water
- 4 green tea bags
- 2 tsp. of honey

Instructions

- In a pan, add the strips & water. Let it come to a boil, turn the heat low.
- Simmer for 10 minutes. Take the strips out.
- Add the tea bags, cover & steep as per the package instructions. Discard the tea bags & mix in honey.
- Serve with a slice of lemon.

Nutrition: Kcal 16| Protein 0.2 g | Fiber 0.6 g | Carbs 5 g | Fat 0.2 g

4. Lemon Tea W/ Honey & Ginger

(Prep time: 10 minutes | Servings: 1)

Ingredients

- Hot water, as need
- Honey, to taste
- 2 to 3 tbsp. of lemon juice
- Fresh chopped ginger, to taste

Instructions

- In a pan, add water & heat.
- Add the rest of the ingredients to the mug.
- Pour hot water & stir, serve.

Nutrition: Kcal 54 | Protein 0.2 g | Fiber 0.2 g | Carbs 14 g | Fat 0.2 g

5. Healthy Sweet Tea

(Prep time: 10 minutes | Servings: 8)

Ingredients

- 4 cups of cold water
- 1/3 cup of raw honey
- 8 tea bags (green or black)
- 4 cups of boiling water

Instructions

- In a pitcher, add the hot water & tea bags. Let them steep for 15 minutes.
- Take the tea bags out & discard them. Add the rest of the ingredients. Mix well & serve.

Nutrition: Kcal 34 | Protein 0 g | Fiber 0.1 g | Carbs 9 g | Fat 0.2 g

6. Sinus Clearing Tea

(Prep time: 10 minutes / Servings: 1)

Ingredients

- 2 tbsp. of Pure Honey
- ¼ cup of Lemon Juice/apple cider vinegar
- ¾ cup of Herbal Tea
- Cayenne pepper, to taste
- Hot Water, as needed

Instructions

- In a pitcher, add hot water & tea, steep as per the package instructions.
- Strain & add the rest of the ingredients.
- Mix & serve.

Nutrition: Kcal 60 | Protein 0.1 g | Fiber 1.2 g | Carbs 18.7 g | Fat 0.2 g

7. Peach Iced Tea

(Prep time: 30 minutes | Cook time: 10 minutes |Servings: 4)

Ingredients

- 1 tea sachet (Earl Grey)
- 4 cups of ice
- 2 cups of water
- 2 tea sachets (English breakfast)

Peach Syrup

- 2 tbsp. of white sugar
- 1 ½ cups of water
- 1 ½ cups of diced peaches

Instructions

- Steep the teas as per package instructions. Discard the tea bags & cool them in the fridge for half an hour.
- In a blender, add all the ingredients of peach syrup. Pulse until chopped.
- Add to a pan heat for 5 minutes. Strain into the tea mix well & serve.

Nutrition: Kcal 51 | Protein 1 g | Fiber 1 g | Carbs 13 g | Fat 1 g

8. Homemade Iced Tea

(Prep time: 20 minutes | Servings: 8)

Ingredients

- 6 cups of boiling water
- 2 cups of fresh herbs
- 8 tea bags
- 4 cups of clear juice

Instructions

- Steep the tea bags in boiling water. Take the tea bags out & add the rest of the ingredients.
- Let it rest for 20 minutes. Strain & serve.

Nutrition: Kcal 57 | Protein 0.1 g | Fiber 1.2 g | Carbs 14 g | Fat 0.2 g

9. Fruit-Infused Iced Green Tea

(Prep time: 20 minutes | Cook time: 5 minutes |Servings: 8)

Ingredients

- 4 ½ cups of boiling water
- 3 peaches, sliced thin
- 2 tbsp. of honey
- 4 green tea bags
- 1 cup of blueberries

Instructions
- In a pitcher, steep tea in boiling water for 5 minutes, discard tea bags.
- Add honey & mix. Add fruits & let them rest for 10 minutes.
- Strain & serve.

Nutrition: Kcal 72 | Protein 0.1 g | Fiber 1.2 g | Carbs 18.7 g | Fat 0.2 g

10. Lemon Ginger Detox Tea

(Prep time: 20 minutes | Cook time: 5 minutes |Servings: 1-2)

Ingredients
- ¼ tsp. of turmeric
- 2 cups of water
- 1 inch of peeled ginger, sliced thin
- ¼ tsp. of maple syrup
- 1 lemon
- Cayenne pepper, a pinch

Instructions
- In a pan, add all ingredients. Mix & heat until it starts to steam.
- Turn the heat off & steep for 5 minutes.
- Strain & serve.

Nutrition: Kcal 12 | Protein 0.3 g | Fiber 0.6 g | Carbs 2.8 g | Fat 0.2 g

11. Moroccan Tea

(Prep time: 10 minutes / Servings: 1)

Ingredients
- 1 tsp. of ground ginger
- Half tsp. of lemon juice
- 1 ½ cups of boiling water
- 1 to 2 tsp. of honey

Instructions
- Add all ingredients in a mug.
- Mix well & serve.

Nutrition: Kcal 28| Protein 0.2 g | Fiber 0.3 g | Carbs 7 g | Fat 0.2 g

12. Fruit-Flavored Iced Green Tea

(Prep time: 15 minutes / Servings: 6)

Ingredients
- 1 lime, sliced thin
- 8 oz. of strawberries, trimmed
- 8 Green Tea Bags
- Zest of 1 lime
- 2 cups of sugar-free non-pulp Orange Juice
- 8 cups of boiling water

Instructions
- Steep the tea in boiling water. Take the tea bags out & keep the tea in the fridge.
- Chop the strawberries in a blender add them to a bowl. Mix with the rest of the ingredients.
- Pour into ice cube tray, freeze for 2 hours.
- Pour tea in a glass with fruit ice cubes. Strain & serve.

Nutrition: Kcal 72 | Protein 0.1 g | Fiber 1.2 g | Carbs 7 g | Fat 0.2 g

13. Melon Honey Green Tea

(Prep time: 15 minutes | Servings: 2)

Ingredients
- 1 bottle of Honey Green Tea (not sweet)
- 6 chunks of honeydew melon, cut into small squares
- 15 fresh mint leaves

Instructions

- In a bowl, add all ingredients & crush with a spoon.
- Mix well & strain. Serve with ice.

Nutrition: Kcal 72 | Protein 0.1 g | Fiber 1.1 g | Carbs 11 g | Fat 0.2 g

14. Southern Sweet Iced Tea

(Prep time: 15 minutes / Servings: 4)

Ingredients

- Half cup of honey
- 8 cups of water
- 4 black tea bags

Instructions

- Steep the tea bags in boiling water for 5 minutes.
- Discard the tea bags add the rest of the ingredients.
- Stir well & serve.

Nutrition: Kcal 98 | Protein 0.3 g | Fiber 0.2 g | Carbs 11 g | Fat 0.2 g

15. Ginger Root Tea

(Prep time: 15 minutes | Cook time: 10 minutes | Servings: 2)

Ingredients

- 1 tsp. of honey
- 4 thin slices of lemon
- 2 cups of water
- 2" piece of peeled ginger, sliced
- 12 mint leaves

Instructions

- Boil water, add ginger & lemon. Steep for a few minutes.
- Add mint leaves & simmer for ten minutes.
- Turn the heat off, add honey. Mix & strain, serve.

Nutrition: Kcal 54 | Protein 0.2 g | Fiber 0.3 g | Carbs 13 g | Fat 0.1 g

16. Citrus Green Tea

(Prep time: 15 minutes | Servings: 2)

Ingredients

- 6 green tea bags
- 4 packets stevia
- 1 lemon & 1 lime, cut into wedges
- 4 cups of water
- 1 orange, cut into wedges

Instructions

- Steep the tea bags in boiling water for 15 minutes.
- Cool & keep in the fridge after adding the rest of the ingredients.
- Strain & serve chilled

Nutrition: Kcal 0 | Protein 0 g | Fiber 0 g | Carbs 0 g | Fat 0 g

17. Iced Green Tea

(Prep time: 15 minutes | Servings: 3)

Ingredients

- Fresh mint leaves
- 3 green tea bags
- 1 lemon, thinly sliced
- 2 cups of boiling water

Instructions

- Steep the tea in boiling water, discard tea bags & add to a pot.
- Cool slightly & add lemon slices.
- Add mint leaves let it rest for a few minutes. Serve.

Nutrition: Kcal 0 | Protein 0 g | Fiber 0 g | Carbs 0 g | Fat 0 g

18. Apple Iced tea

(Prep time: 15 minutes | Servings: 3)

Ingredients

- 4 cups of water

- 1 lemon, thinly sliced
- 2 cinnamon sticks
- 4 cups of clear apple juice
- 2 tea bags (English breakfast)
- Honey, to taste
- 1 red apple, thinly sliced

Instructions
- Steep the tea bags in boiling water for 15 minutes. Discard the tea bags add the rest of the ingredients.
- Chill in the fridge & serve.

Nutrition: Kcal 72 | Protein 0.1 g | Fiber 1.2 g | Carbs 18.7 g | Fat 0.2 g

19. The All Fix Tea

(Prep time: 15 minutes | Servings: 1)

Ingredients
- 1 tbsp. of honey
- 1" of sliced fresh ginger
- 1 small stick of cinnamon
- 1 sliced clove of garlic
- Juice of half lemon

Instructions
- In a cheesecloth, add the garlic, cinnamon & ginger. Wrap them tightly.
- Add to a mug with the rest of the ingredients. Steep for 8 minutes.
- Take the cheesecloth out & serve.

Nutrition: Kcal 65 | Protein 0.1 g | Fiber 1 g | Carbs 11 g | Fat 0.2 g

20. Immune Boon Herbal Tea

(Prep time: 35 minutes | Servings: 1)

Ingredients
- 1 tbsp. of dried elderberries
- 1 tbsp. of dried echinacea flowers & leaves
- 1 tbsp. of dried ginger root

- 1 tbsp. of dried rose hips
- 1 tbsp. of dried astragalus

Instructions
- In an air-tight jar, add all the ingredients. Mix & keep in a cool, dry place.
- To make one cup of tea, add 1 tbsp. of the mixture in a mug, add boiling water & steep for half an hour or more.
- Strain, add honey to your taste. Serve.

Nutrition: Kcal 65| Protein 0.2 g | Fiber 1.1 g | Carbs 11 g | Fat 0.2 g

21. NyQuell Herbal Tea

(Prep time: 35 minutes | Servings: 1-2)

Ingredients
- 1 tbsp. of dried valerian root
- 1 tbsp. of dried peppermint leaf
- 1 tbsp. of dried chamomile flower
- 1 tbsp. of dried licorice root

Instructions
- In an air-tight jar, add all the ingredients. Mix & keep in a cool, dry place.
- To make one cup of tea, add 1 tbsp. of the mixture in a mug, add boiling water & steep for half an hour or more.
- Strain, add honey to your taste. Serve.

Nutrition: Kcal 67 | Protein 0.1 g | Fiber 1.1 g | Carbs 11 g | Fat 0.3 g

22. Healthy Fruit Juice

(Prep time: 15 minutes | Servings: 1-2)

Ingredients
- 1 cup of grapefruit, peeled
- 2 tbsp. of lemon juice
- 1 tbsp. of honey

- Half cup of ice cubes
- 1 cup of pomegranate seeds
- Half cup of water
- 1 orange

Instructions
- In a blender, add all the fruits with the rest of the ingredients.
- Strain the juice & serve.

Nutrition: Kcal 77 | Protein 0.8 g | Fiber 1.6 g | Carbs 10 g | Fat 1.2 g

23. Green Goddess Juice

(Prep time: 15 minutes | Servings: 1-2)

Ingredients
- 1 pear, cut into 8 wedges
- Half cucumber, slice into fours
- 3 celery stalks
- 1 green apple, cut into 8 wedges

Instructions
- In a blender, add all the fruits with enough water.
- Strain the juice & serve.

Nutrition: Kcal 74| Protein 0.1 g | Fiber 1.4 g | Carbs 12 g | Fat 1.3 g

24. Pineapple juice

(Prep time: 15 minutes | Servings: 6)

Ingredients
- 1 cup of water
- ¼ tsp. of black pepper & salt (optional)
- 2 cups of pineapple cubes
- Half" of peeled ginger

Instructions
- In a blender, add all the ingredients.
- Pulse until smooth strain & serve chilled.

Nutrition: Kcal 76 | Protein 0.2 g | Fiber 1.1 g | Carbs 12 g | Fat 0.2 g

25. Ginger Zinger Juice

(Prep time: 15 minutes | Servings: 6)

Ingredients
- ¼ lemon, peeled
- 5 carrots
- 2 apples, sliced thin
- Half" of fresh ginger

Instructions
- In a blender, add all the ingredients.
- Pulse until smooth strain & serve chilled.

Nutrition: Kcal 78 | Protein 0.7 g | Fiber 1.6 g | Carbs 11.9 g | Fat 0.3 g

26. Beet Juice

(Prep time: 15 minutes | Servings: 4)

Ingredients
- 2 green apples, diced
- 2 beets, washed & trimmed
- 1 juice of 1 lemon
- 2 carrots, chopped
- 2 cups of water
- 2 peeled clementines
- 7 strawberries, trimmed
- 1" piece of fresh peeled ginger

Instructions
- In a blender, add all the ingredients.
- Pulse until smooth, strain & serve chilled.

Nutrition: Kcal 87| Protein 0.1 g | Fiber 1.4 g | Carbs 14.6 g | Fat 0.3 g

27. Iced Green Tea with Mint & Ginger

(Prep time: 15 minutes | Cook time: 10 minutes |Servings: 4)

Ingredients
- ¼ cup of peeled ginger, sliced
- 1/3 cup of honey
- 3-6 green tea bags

- 1 lemon, divided
- 6 cups of water
- Half cup of mint leaves

Instructions
- In a pot, add ginger & water. Let it come to a boil, add mint & teabags. Steep for 15 minutes.
- Strain & add honey.
- Serve chilled.

Nutrition: Kcal 75 | Protein 0.1 g | Fiber 1.2 g | Carbs 18.7 g | Fat 0.2 g

28. Strawberry-Basil Iced Tea

(Prep time: 35 minutes | Cook time: 10 minutes |Servings: 8)

Ingredients
- Ice, for serving
- 1 pound of strawberries, trimmed & cut into fours
- 1 cup of fresh basil
- 4 cups of water or more
- 8 black-tea bags
- 3/4 cup of sugar

Instructions
- In a pan, add water and boil. Add tea bags & steep for 5 minutes.
- In a separate pot, add sugar & water. Stir well on low heat & cook until sugar dissolves.
- Turn the heat off & add basil. Let it rest for 10 minutes.
- Add to the strawberries & toss well. Let it rest for 25 minutes.
- Add the tea to the strawberries let it rest for a few hours in the fridge.
- Serve chilled after straining.

Nutrition: Kcal 79 | Protein 0.1 g | Fiber 1 g | Carbs 19 g | Fat 0.2 g

29. Hibiscus-Mint Iced Tea

(Prep time: 15 minutes | Cook time: 10 minutes |Servings: 8)

Ingredients
- 4 cups of boiling water
- 4 hibiscus tea bags
- 2 cups of cold water
- Half cup of fresh mint leaves
- 2 cups of apple juice

Instructions
- In a pot, add mint leaves, tea bags & boiling water. Let it rest for 10 minutes.
- Take the mint & tea bags out. Add cold water & apple juice. Mix well & serve.

Nutrition: Kcal 81 | Protein 1 g | Fiber 1.3 g | Carbs 12 g | Fat 0.2 g

30. Pineapple Skin Tea

(Prep time: 15 minutes | Cook time: 10 minutes |Servings: 16)

Ingredients
- 1 pineapple, peel & core
- 3 tbsp. of grated ginger
- 2 oranges
- 17 cups of water
- 2 tbsp. of grated turmeric
- Half tsp. of Cayenne pepper
- 3 tbsp. of honey
- 2 sprigs of herbs
- 1 lemon
- 2 cinnamon sticks

Instructions
- Clean the pineapple skin thoroughly. Add to a large pan, add 1-2 tbsp. of vinegar.
- Soak for half an hour & rinse well. Pat dry & peel & core with a knife.

- In a pot, add all ingredients (do not add honey yet), mix & place on a medium flame.
- Simmer for half an hour or more. Strain & add to the pitcher.
- Serve with the desired amount of honey.

Nutrition: Kcal 55 | Protein 1 g | Fiber 1.2 g | Carbs 14 g | Fat 1 g

31. Lemon-Rosemary Iced Tea

(Prep time: 25 minutes | Cook time: 15 minutes |Servings: 4)

Ingredients

- 1 cup of lemon juice
- 2 cups of sugar
- 5 cups of water
- 12 sprigs of fresh rosemary
- 1/4 cup of black tea leaves

Instructions

- In a pan, add herbs, sugar & water. Simmer until sugar dissolves.
- Turn the heat off. Add tea leaves & steep for 3 minutes.
- Strain & serve with lemon juice.

Nutrition: Kcal 401 | Protein 1 g | Fiber 1 g | Carbs 104 g | Fat 1 g

32. Watermelon Juice

(Prep time: 25 minutes | Servings: 4)

Ingredients

- 3 lime wedges
- 4 cups of watermelon cubes
- 1 cup of ice
- 1-2 tbsp. of sugar
- Half tsp. of sea salt

Instructions

- Add all ingredients to a blender. Pulse until smooth.
- Strain & serve.

Nutrition: Kcal 96 | Protein 2 g | Fiber 3 g | Carbs 26 g | Fat 1 g

33. Antioxidant Blast Juice

(Prep time: 25 minutes | Servings: 4)

Ingredients

- 2 beets, trimmed & cut into wedges
- 1 cup of blueberries
- 1 cup of strawberries, halved
- Water, as needed

Instructions

- Add all ingredients to a blender. Pulse until smooth.
- Strain & serve.

Nutrition: Kcal 76| Protein 1.3 g | Fiber 0.4 g | Carbs 12 g | Fat 0.3 g

34. Pear Juice

(Prep time: 15 minutes | Servings: 1)

Ingredients

- Water, as needed
- 1 Pear, peeled & cut

Instructions

- Add all ingredients to a blender. Pulse until smooth.
- Strain & serve.

Nutrition: Kcal 34| Protein 0.7 g | Fiber 1.0 g | Carbs 14 g | Fat 0.2 g

35. Cucumber Cooler Juice

(Prep time: 15 minutes | Servings: 1)

Ingredients

- 1/4 of a peeled lemon
- 2 stalks of celery
- 1/4 of a cantaloupe, peeled & cut into pieces
- Half cucumber, sliced thin

Instructions

- Add all ingredients to a blender. Pulse until smooth.

- Strain & serve.

Nutrition: Kcal 69 | Protein 0.1 g | Fiber 1.2 g | Carbs 13 g | Fat 0.2 g

36. Cucumber Limeade

(Prep time: 15 minutes | Servings: 1)

Ingredients

- 3 limes' juice
- 1 peeled cucumber, cut into pieces
- Half or 1 cup of simple syrup
- Water, as needed

Instructions

- Add all ingredients to a blender. Pulse until smooth.
- Strain & serve with ice.

Nutrition: Kcal 56| Protein 0.1 g | Fiber 1 g | Carbs 13 g | Fat 0.2 g

38. Green Smoothie Popsicles

(Prep time: 4 hours & 15 minutes / Servings: 2-4)

Ingredients

- 2 cups of coconut water or more
- 1 tbsp. of grated ginger
- 4 tbsp. of honey
- ¼ cup of parsley
- 1 cup of fresh spinach
- 2 kiwis, peeled

Instructions

- Add all ingredients to a blender. Pulse until smooth.
- Strain well & pour in the molds. Keep in the freezer until they set.
- Serve.

Nutrition: Kcal 45 | Protein 1 g | Fiber 0.8 g | Carbs 10 g | Fat 5.3 g

39. Blackberry-Rose Ice Pops

(Prep time: 4 hours & 15 minutes | Cook time: 10 minutes |Servings: 10)

Ingredients

- 5 cups of blackberries
- 3 cups of coconut water
- 1 tsp. of rosewater
- 1 tbsp. of lemon juice
- 9 tbsp. of cane sugar

Instructions

- Add sugar & the same amount of water in a pan. Stir on medium flame until dissolved.
- Add the rest of the ingredients to a blender pulse until smooth.
- Strain & mix with the syrup. Pour in the molds. Keep in the freezer until they set.
- Serve.

Nutrition: Kcal 45 | Protein 0.8 g | Fiber 0.8 g | Carbs 11 g | Fat 5.3 g

4.2 LUNCH & DINNER

1. Basic Bone Broth

(Prep time: 15 minutes | Cook time: 12 hours & 20 minutes | Servings: 8)

Ingredients

- 1 onion, roughly chopped
- 3 garlic cloves
- 2 celery stalks, roughly chopped
- Water, as needed
- 2 Pounds of beef bones
- Half tbsp. of peppercorns
- 2 carrots, roughly chopped
- 2 bay leaves
- 2 tbsp. of apple cider vinegar
- 1 tbsp. of salt

Instructions

- Add all ingredients to a large pot with water to cover the beef bones.
- Let it come to a boil simmer for 12 hours on low. Keep adding water & skim the foam on top.
- Cool & strain. Serve.

Nutrition: Kcal 78 | Protein 6 g | Fiber 1.0 g | Carbs 11 g | Fat 0.2 g

2. Clear vegetable soup

(Prep time: 15 minutes | Cook time: 30minutes | Servings: 3)

Ingredients

- 1 yellow onion, chopped
- 1 cup of cauliflower florets
- 2 carrots, roughly chopped
- 1 ½ cups of sliced mushrooms
- 12 French beans
- 1 cup of chopped celery stalks
- 1 cup of spring onion
- Water, as needed

Instructions

- In a pot, add all ingredients. Add enough water to cover the vegetables.
- Simmer on a medium flame for 30 minutes. Add more water if needed.
- Strain & add salt pepper. Serve.

Nutrition: Kcal 141 | Protein 5 g | Fiber 5 g | Carbs 19 g | Fat 5 g

3. Chicken Clear Soup

(Prep time: 15 minutes | Cook time: 30 minutes | Servings: 4)

Ingredients

- ¼ cup of chopped onion
- 4 cups of water
- 3 to 4 smashed garlic cloves
- 2 to 3 sprigs of thyme
- ¼ cup of chopped carrot
- 10.5 oz. of chicken with bones
- ¼ tsp. of black pepper
- 2 bay leaves
- Salt, to taste

Instructions

- Wash the chicken with bones.
- Add all the ingredients to a pressure cooker. Cook on high heat for 1 whistle.
- Turn the heat low & simmer for 10 to 12 minutes.
- Turn the heat off release the pressure naturally.
- Strain & serve.

Nutrition: Kcal 172 | Protein 14 g | Fiber 3 g | Carbs 2 g | Fat 11 g

4. Vegetable Chicken Clear Soup

(Prep time: 15 minutes | Cook time: 30 minutes |Servings: 1)

Ingredients

- 1-inch piece of ginger
- 1/4 cup of peas
- Half capsicum
- 2 Cloves of garlic
- 2 pieces of chicken (bone-in)
- 1 carrot
- Half tsp. of Black pepper
- Half cup of cabbage
- Salt, to taste

Instructions

- Add garlic, chicken, water & ginger to a pan. Cook till it is done.
- Strain & add vegetables. Cook for 10 minutes more.
- Strain & serve.

Nutrition: Kcal 65 | Protein 3 g | Fiber 1.2 g | Carbs 10 g | Fat 1.2 g

5. Garlic Chicken Soup

(Prep time: 15 minutes | Cook time: 20 minutes |Servings: 2)

Ingredients

- 2 lemon wedges
- 3.5 oz. of chicken, thinly sliced
- 2 garlic cloves, thinly sliced
- Salt & pepper to taste
- 2 tsp. of sesame oil
- 6 cups of water
- 1 large carrot, cut into strips
- 3 scallions, diced

Instructions

- Sauté garlic in a drizzle of oil until crispy.
- Add the rest of the ingredients with water.

- Let it come to a boil simmer for 2 to 3 minutes. Strain & serve.

Nutrition: Kcal 82 | Protein 2 g | Fiber 0.3 g | Carbs 11 g | Fat 4 g

6. Japanese Clear Soup

(Prep time: 15 minutes | Cook time: 1 hour & 10 minutes |Servings: 2)

Ingredients

- 8 cups of chicken broth
- 6 smashed cloves garlic, peeled
- 4 cups of beef broth
- 4 cups of water
- 2 tsp. of sesame oil
- 4 scallions, diced
- 1 yellow onion, roughly sliced
- 10 button mushrooms, thinly sliced
- 2 large carrots, cut into chunks
- 2" piece of ginger, sliced
- Salt, to taste

Instructions

- In a stock pot, sauté carrots, onion, ginger & garlic in a drizzle of oil for a few minutes.
- Add water, beef broth & chicken broth. Let it come to a boil, turn the heat low and simmer for 60 minutes.
- Strain & add salt pepper. Serve.

Nutrition: Kcal 46 | Protein 3 g | Fiber 0 g | Carbs 7 g | Fat 1 g

7. Healthy Chicken Soup

(Prep time: 15 minutes | Cook time: 30 minutes |Servings: 4)

Ingredients

- 2 Thyme sprigs
- ½ cup of Corn Kernels
- 1 Carrot
- 2 tbsp. of Light Soy Sauce
- ½ Chicken

- 1 Onion
- ½ Lemongrass
- ½ cup of Peas
- 2 Garlic Cloves
- 6 cups of Water
- Salt to Taste

Instructions

- In a large pot, add all ingredients with enough water to cover the ingredients.
- Simmer for 45 minutes.
- Strain & adjust seasoning. Serve.

Nutrition: Kcal 66 | Protein 2 g | Fiber 1.1 g | Carbs 11 g | Fat 2 g

8. Easy Miso Soup

(Prep time: 15 minutes | Cook time: 20 minutes |Servings: 10)

Ingredients

- 1/3 cup seaweed
- 1 cup of scallions, chopped
- 3 sheets of nori
- 8 cups of water
- ½ cup of white miso paste
- 1 cup of mushrooms
- 2 cups of baby spinach
- 7 oz. of silken tofu, cubed

Instructions

- In a pot, add water & boil. Add all the ingredients except for miso paste.
- Cook for 5-7 minutes. Take some water out & mix with miso, add back to the soup.
- Cook for a few minutes. Strain & Serve.

Nutrition: Kcal 64 | Protein 4 g | Fiber 2 g | Carbs 9 g | Fat 1 g

9. Leeks Clear Soup

(Prep time: 15 minutes | Cook time: 20 minutes |Servings: 2)

Ingredients

- 4 to 5 cloves of Garlic
- 1 tbsp. of olive oil
- 1 cup of chopped Leeks
- 1 cup of chicken with bones
- Salt & black pepper, to taste
- 4 cups of Water

Instructions

- Sauté the garlic for 30 seconds in hot oil. Add leeks & mushrooms, sauté for 2 to 3 minutes.
- Add the rest of the ingredients.
- Simmer for 10 to 15 minutes. Strain & serve.

Nutrition: Kcal 72 | Protein 0.1 g | Fiber 1.2 g | Carbs 18.7 g | Fat 0.2 g

10. Chicken Broth

(Prep time: 15 minutes | Cook time: 20 minutes |Servings: 8)

Ingredients

- 1 onion, cut into fours
- 2 carrots, roughly chopped
- 1 parsnip, peeled & chopped
- 2 stalks celery, roughly chopped
- 3 sprigs of parsley
- 4 pounds of whole chicken
- 5 black peppercorns
- 1 leek, chopped
- 16 cups of water
- 3 sprigs of fresh thyme
- 1 bay leaf

Instructions

- Add all ingredients to a large pot.
- Let it come to a boil, turn the heat low and simmer for 1 hour.
- Strain & adjust seasoning.

- Serve.

Nutrition: Kcal 71 | Protein 2 g | Fiber 1.3 g | Carbs 11 g | Fat 1.2 g

11. Crab, Tomato & Fennel Broth

(Prep time: 15 minutes | Cook time: 30 minutes |Servings: 4)

Ingredients

- 1 fennel bulb, sliced
- 1 onion, sliced
- 4 crab claws, split
- 4 plum tomatoes, chopped without seeds
- Salt & black pepper, to taste
- 1 garlic clove, chopped
- 2 celery stalks, chopped
- 1 cup of small fennel fronds
- Splash of white wine
- 5.3 oz. of white crab meat

Instructions

- Sauté the crab claws in hot oil for on high heat for a few minutes.
- Add the rest of the vegetables (except for tomatoes) cook for 6 to 7 minutes.
- Add wine & deglaze. Add 4 cups of water, boil & simmer for 20 minutes.
- Add crab meat & tomatoes. Season to taste.
- Strain & serve.

Nutrition: Kcal 87 | Protein 3 g | Fiber 1 g | Carbs 12 g | Fat 6 g

12. Chicken Bone Broth

(Prep time: 15 minutes | Cook time: 20 minutes |Servings: 4)

Ingredients

- 2 tbsp. of oil
- ½ cup of green part scallions
- 1 chicken, cut into pieces
- 2 carrots, chopped

- 5 peppercorns
- 2 parsnips, chopped
- 8 cups water
- 1 celery stalk, chopped
- Half tsp. of salt

Instructions

- Sauté the scallions for 2-3 minutes in hot oil. Add the rest of the ingredients.
- Let it come to a boil, turn the heat low and simmer for 2 & a half hours.
- Strain & adjust seasoning. Serve.

Nutrition: Kcal 82 | Protein 3 g | Fiber 1 g | Carbs 13 g | Fat 4.2 g

13. Oxtail Soup

(Prep time: 15 minutes | Cook time: 3 hours |Servings: 4)

Ingredients

- 2 shallots, chopped
- ½ leek, chopped
- 1 carrot, chopped
- 1 tsp. of Marmite
- 1 oxtail cut
- 1 tsp. of Worcestershire sauce
- 1 stick of celery, chopped
- 1 garlic clove, chopped
- 1 tbsp. of dark sugar
- 1 tsp. of tomato puree
- 4 sprigs thyme
- 4 cups of chicken stock
- 2 bay leaves

Instructions

- Sauté the oxtail on high flame in a splash of hot oil until seared.
- Add the rest of the ingredients simmer for 2 to 3 hours.
- Strain & adjust seasoning. Serve.

Nutrition: Kcal 88 | Protein 5 g | Fiber 1 g | Carbs 17 g | Fat 1.8 g

14. Mutton Soup

(Prep time: 15 minutes | Cook time: 1 hour & 10 minutes |Servings: 4)

Ingredients

- 1 garlic clove
- 4 black peppercorn
- Salt & black pepper, to taste
- 7 oz. of Mutton with bone
- 4 to 5 cups of water
- 1"cinnamon stick
- ½ tsp. of oil

Instructions

- Sauté the cinnamon, peppercorn & clove in hot oil for a few seconds.
- Add mutton cook until it is seared.
- Add the rest of the ingredients. Cook for 60 minutes.
- Adjust seasoning & strain. Serve.

Nutrition: Kcal 76 | Protein 5 g | Fiber 0.5 g | Carbs 11 g | Fat 5.2 g

15. Simple Vegetable Broth

(Prep time: 15 minutes | Cook time: 1 hour & 10 minutes |Servings: 4)

Ingredients

- 1 ear corn
- ½ cup of scallions, chopped
- 2 parsnips, chopped
- ½ cup of leeks, chopped
- 8 cups of water
- ½ tsp. of salt & pepper, each
- 2 carrots, chopped
- 1 bay leaf
- 1 celery stalk
- 1 tbsp. of garlic-infused oil

Instructions

- In a pan, add all ingredients except for water.
- Sauté for a few minutes. Add water & cook for half an hour to 60 minutes.
- Adjust seasoning & strain. Serve.

Nutrition: Kcal 77 | Protein 3 g | Fiber 1 g | Carbs 13.2 g | Fat 0.9 g

16. Shellfish Broth

(Prep time: 15 minutes | Cook time: 1 hour & 10 minutes |Servings: 8-12)

Ingredients

- ½ cup of dry white wine
- 1 celery stalk, chopped
- 1 yellow onion, chopped
- 4-6 cups of shellfish shells
- 1 bay leaf
- 1 carrot, chopped
- 2 tbsp. of tomato paste
- 10-15 whole peppercorns
- 2 sprigs of thyme
- Several sprigs of parsley
- 2 tsp. of salt

Instructions

- Break the shells. Roast the shells for 10 minutes at 400°F.
- Add to a pan & cover with water. Place on medium heat & do not stir.
- Simmer for an hour. Add the rest of the ingredients.
- Simmer for half an hour. Strain well & adjust seasoning.
- Serve.

Nutrition: Kcal 75 | Protein 4 g | Fiber 1 g | Carbs 12 g | Fat 1.2 g

17. Seafood Broth

(Prep time: 15 minutes | Cook time: 50 minutes |Servings: 4)

Ingredients

- 2 oz. of onion
- 1 tbsp. of chopped garlic
- 1 bay leaf
- 2 oz. of sea bass
- 7.7 oz. of prawn shells
- 2 oz. of prawns
- 2 oz. of squid
- 0.3 oz. of celery
- 2 oz. of tomatoes
- ½ tbsp. of black pepper corns
- Salt, to taste
- 0.3 oz. of leeks
- 2 tbsp olive oil
- 1 oz. of carrot

Instructions
- Roast the prawn shells for 20 minutes at 320°F.
- Sauté vegetables for a few minutes and add the shells.
- Add the rest of the ingredients.
- Cook for 20 minutes. Strain & serve after adjusting seasoning.

Nutrition: Kcal 65 | Protein 4 g | Fiber 0.7 g | Carbs 11 g | Fat 1.2 g

18. Seafood Stew

(Prep time: 15 minutes | Cook time: 60 minutes |Servings: 4)

Ingredients
- 1 shallot, sliced thin
- 1 1/2 cups of chicken stock
- 2 garlic cloves, chopped
- 2 tbsp. of olive oil
- ½ cup of dry white wine
- 1 cup of bottled clam juice
- Canned 1 cup drained tomatoes
- ½ pound of deveined & shelled shrimp
- 1 bay leaf
- 2 thyme sprigs

- ½ tsp. of hot sauce
- Salt and pepper, to taste
- 24 littleneck clams, washed
- 2 tbsp. of chopped parsley
- 3/4 pound of snapper fillets, skinless
- 2 tbsp. of unsalted butter

Instructions
- In a pot, sauté the garlic & shallots in hot oil for 3 minutes.
- Add wine & cook until reduced. Add the rest of the ingredients except for clams, snapper & shrimps.
- Let it come to a boil, turn the heat low. Simmer for 10 minutes.
- Add the rest of the seafood & cook for 5-7 minutes.
- Serve.

Nutrition: Kcal 89 | Protein 7 g | Fiber 1.3 g | Carbs 12.1 g | Fat 5.2 g

19. Sicilian Fish Stew

(Prep time: 15 minutes | Cook time: 30 minutes |Servings: 4)

Ingredients
- 1/4 cup of minced yellow onion
- 1 tbsp. of minced garlic
- 2 tbsp. of chopped seeded tomato
- 1/4 cup of dry vermouth
- 2 tbsp. of olive oil
- 3 cups of Fish Stock
- 2 tbsp. of golden raisins
- 1 tbsp. of drained capers
- ½ tsp. of ground coriander
- 1-2 halibut fillets
- 3 pounds of shrimp

Instructions
- Sauté the vegetables in hot oil on a medium flame for 1 minute.
- Add the vermouth & stock, let it come to a simmer.

- Add fish & shrimp, cook, until done. Add more stock if it is too thick.
- Adjust seasoning & strain. Serve.

Nutrition: Kcal 92 | Protein 5 g | Fiber 1.2 g | Carbs 13 g | Fat 6 g

20. Clear Chicken Soup

(Prep time: 15 minutes | Cook time: 30 minutes |Servings: 4)

Ingredients

- 1 tbsp. of butter
- 2 cups of chicken with bones
- Water, as needed
- 2 scallions
- Salt, to taste
- 2 egg
- Black pepper, to taste

Instructions

- In a pan, melt butter. Sauté the spring onion till it browns.
- Add chicken & cook until it browns.
- In a large pan, add water & boil. Add the chicken mixture.
- Let it simmer for half an hour.
- Strain & adjust seasoning. Add the whisked egg whites while stirring
- Add salt & pepper, cook for 2 minutes. Strain & serve.

Nutrition: Kcal 89| Protein 4 g | Fiber 1.0 g | Carbs 11 g | Fat 0.2 g

21. Clear Onion Soup

(Prep time: 15 minutes | Cook time: 40 minutes |Servings: 6)

Ingredients

- 2 diced onions
- 1 celery stalks, chopped
- 1 cup of sliced button mushrooms
- 1 carrot, diced
- 6 cups vegetable broth
- Salt & pepper, to taste

- ½ tsp. of minced ginger & minced garlic, each
- 1 tsp. of sesame oil
- ½ cup of scallions

Instructions

- In a pot, sauté the onion for 10 minutes until slightly caramelized.
- Add the rest of the ingredients simmer for half an hour.
- Strain & adjust seasoning. Serve.

Nutrition: Kcal 24 | Protein 2 g | Fiber 1 g | Carbs 2 g | Fat 1 g

22. Hibachi Clear Soup

(Prep time: 15 minutes | Cook time: 90 minutes |Servings: 8)

Ingredients

- 1 onion, diced
- 3" ginger, peeled & chopped
- 4 cups of water
- 1 carrot, chopped
- 1 tbsp. of sesame oil
- 4 cups of beef broth
- 4 minced cloves garlic
- 8 cups of chicken broth

Instructions

- Sauté the vegetables in hot oil for a few minutes.
- Add all the liquids & boil.
- Simmer for 60 minutes. Strain & serve.

Nutrition: Kcal 55 | Protein 3 g | Fiber 1.2 g | Carbs 6.1 g | Fat 2.3 g

23. Mushroom Clear Soup

(Prep time: 15 minutes | Cook time: 40 minutes |Servings: 2)

Ingredients

- 4 cups of water
- 7 oz. of button mushrooms, cleaned & sliced
- 1 tbsp. butter
- Few sprigs Thyme
- 1 tsp. of salt

Instructions

- Sauté the mushrooms in butter for a few seconds.
- Add the rest of the ingredients.
- Simmer for half an hour. Strain & adjust seasoning.
- Serve.

Nutrition: Kcal 72 | Protein 0.1 g | Fiber 1.2 g | Carbs 11 g | Fat 0.2 g

24. Big, Clear Vegetable Soup

(Prep time: 15 minutes | Cook time: 40 minutes |Servings: 4)

Ingredients

- 1 tbsp. of fish sauce
- ¼ of a Chinese cabbage
- 1 tbsp. of soy sauce
- 1 tbsp. of sake
- 1 cup of dried shiitake mushrooms
- 1 tbsp. of mirin
- salt, to season
- 1 sweet potato, peeled and chopped
- 3 scallions, sliced
- 1 tbsp. of vegetable oil
- 1 tsp. of sesame oil
- 2 carrots, peeled and chopped
- 10 oz. of firm tofu, cubed
- ½ daikon, peeled and chopped

Instructions

- In a pot, add washed mushrooms with 6 cups of boiling water. Let it rest for 20 minutes.

- Take the mushroom out & trim the stalks; cut the caps in half.
- In the liquid, add the mirin, fish sauce, sake & soy sauce.
- Sauté the vegetables in a different pan in hot oil for 2 minutes.
- Add to the stock & simmer for 15 minutes.
- Add tofu & simmer for 10 minutes. Adjust seasoning, strain & serve.

Nutrition: Kcal 52 | Protein 2 g | Fiber 1 g | Carbs 8.0 g | Fat 4.2 g

25. Light & Delicious Seafood Soup

(Prep time: 15 minutes | Cook time: 40 minutes |Servings: 6)

Ingredients

- 2 tbsp. of olive oil
- 1 white onion, chopped
- 2 celery ribs, chopped
- 1 leek without the dark green part
- Salt and black pepper
- 2 cloves garlic, minced
- 1 pound of deveined & peeled shrimps
- 1 fennel bulb, sliced
- 1 tbsp. of lemon juice
- 5 cups of chicken broth
- 2 tsp. of dried oregano
- ¼ cup of chopped parsley
- Half tsp. of crushed red pepper flakes
- 1 pound scallops, trimmed
- 8 oz. of vegetable stock
- 2 bay leaves
- 2 tsp. of fresh thyme, chopped
- 1 pound of clams

Instructions

- Wash the leek.
- In a Dutch oven, add the butter on a medium flame.

- Sauté the onion, fennel, celery & leek with salt & pepper for 8-10 minutes.
- Add the garlic, pepper flakes & herbs sauté for 1 minute.
- Add bay leaves broths & simmer for 10 minutes.
- Add sea food & simmer for 5-10 minutes.
- Strain & adjust seasoning. Serve.

Nutrition: Kcal 82 | Protein 6 g | Fiber 1.6 g | Carbs 17 g | Fat 7.2 g

26. Clear Fish Soup

(Prep time: 15 minutes | Cook time: 40 minutes |Servings: 4)

Ingredients
- 2 celery stalks
- 25 oz. of fish (mixed)
- 4 carrots
- 6 potatoes
- 1 onion
- Salt & pepper, to taste
- 2 tomatoes
- 2 tbsp. of oil
- 1 bay leaf

Instructions
- Clean the fish add to a pot.
- Add enough water & salt. Boil until half cooked.
- Take the fish out & add the vegetables (peeled & chopped).
- Cook until tender. Strain & serve with a drizzle of lemon juice.

Nutrition: Kcal 65 | Protein 2 g | Fiber 1 g | Carbs 11 g | Fat 1.8 g

27. Seafood Soup with Ginger Broth

(Prep time: 15 minutes | Cook time: 40 minutes |Servings: 4)

Ingredients
- 1 tsp. of olive oil
- 1 tsp. of lemon zest
- 1/4 tsp. of red pepper flakes
- 2 minced garlic cloves
- 4 cups of chicken broth
- 1 tbsp. of soy sauce
- 1 tsp. of sesame oil
- 1 tbsp. of lemon juice
- 4 scallions, chopped
- 1 tbsp. of peeled & minced gingerroot
- 1/4 lb. of peeled & diced shrimp
- 3 carrots, peeled & sliced
- 1/4 lb. of diced scallops

Instructions
- Sauté the ginger, pepper flakes, garlic & lemon zest until fragrant.
- Add lemon juice, broth & soy sauce. Let it come to a boil.
- Add carrots simmer for 15 minutes. Add the rest of the ingredients.
- Cook until done, strain & serve.

Nutrition: Kcal 52 | Protein 3 g | Fiber 1 g | Carbs 11 g | Fat 1.6 g

28. Fish & Shrimp Broth

(Prep time: 15 minutes | Cook time: 40 minutes |Servings: 4)

Ingredients
- 17 oz. of fish
- 2 onions
- 1 tbsp. of vegetable oil
- ½ cup of dry vermouth
- 4 cups of water
- 1 tsp. of coriander
- 8 oz. of raw shrimp, without shells
- 1 bay leaf
- 1 bunch of dill
- 1 ½ cups of white wine
- 2 fennel bulb
- 2 carrots

- Salt & pepper, to taste

Instructions

- Sauté the chopped onion, bay leaf, shrimps & coriander seeds in hot oil for a few minutes.
- Add vermouth, fish, water & wine. Boil & simmer for 20 minutes.
- Strain the broth, add peeled & chopped vegetables with shrimp. Cook until done.
- Adjust seasoning. Strain & serve.

Nutrition: Kcal 69.7 | Protein 3 g | Fiber 1 g | Carbs 11 g | Fat 3.2 g

29. Clear Tomato Broth

(Prep time: 15 minutes | Cook time: 70 minutes |Servings: 4)

Ingredients

- 1 onion
- Salt, to taste
- 4 cups of beef broth
- 4 black peppercorns
- 1 pinch of sugar
- 3 egg whites
- 28 oz. of tomatoes
- ½ tsp. of dried tarragon
- 2 carrots
- 1 bay leaf
- 2 oz. snow peas

Instructions

- Peel & chop the vegetables. Whisk egg whites.
- In a pot, add all ingredients. Simmer for 1 hour.
- Strain well, serve.

Nutrition: Kcal 66 | Protein 2 g | Fiber 1 g | Carbs 11 g | Fat 0.2 g

30. Spiced Clear Broth

(Prep time: 15 minutes | Cook time: 40 minutes |Servings: 4)

Ingredients

- 3 stalks of cilantro
- ⅔ cup of peeled & sliced fresh ginger
- Salt & peppers
- 4 cups of vegetable stock
- 1 tbsp. of sesame seeds

Instructions

- In a pot, add all ingredients. Boil & then simmer for 5 minutes.
- Strain & serve.

Nutrition: Kcal 23 | Protein 0 g | Fiber 0 g | Carbs 0 g | Fat 0.2 g

31. Mussel Broth

(Prep time: 15 minutes | Cook time: 40 minutes |Servings: 6)

Ingredients

- 2 scallions, sliced
- 4 cups of fish stock
- 1 pinch of saffron
- 17 cups of mussels
- 2 tbsp. of olive oil
- ⅜ cup of white wine

Instructions

- Sauté the scallion in hot oil for 60 seconds.
- Add mussels with wine place a lid on top. Cook for 5 minutes.
- Add the rest of the ingredients.
- Adjust seasoning, strain & serve.

Nutrition: Kcal 42 | Protein 2 g | Fiber 0 g | Carbs 8 g | Fat 0 g

32. Fish & Vegetable Soup

(Prep time: 15 minutes | Cook time: 40 minutes |Servings: 4)

Ingredients

- 1 tbsp. of butter
- 1 clove garlic, minced
- 3 ½ cups of chicken broth
- ½ tsp. of dried basil
- 1 cup of sliced carrots
- ¼ cup of diced onion
- 1 cup of green beans
- 1 lb. white fish, cubed
- ½ cup of corn
- ½ tsp. of salt
- ¼ tsp. of dried oregano
- 1/8 tsp. of pepper

Instructions
- Sauté onion & garlic in butter for 2-3 minutes.
- Add the rest of the ingredients, except fish. Simmer for 8 minutes.
- Add fish, cook for 5-7 minutes, strain & serve.

Nutrition: Kcal 190 | Protein 25 g | Fiber 1 g | Carbs 11 g | Fat 4 g

33. Vietnamese Canh

(Prep time: 15 minutes | Cook time: 40 minutes |Servings: 2)

Ingredients
- 1/4 white onion, sliced
- 4 cups of water
- Half tsp. of vegetable oil
- 4 oz. of white fish/shrimp, chopped
- 1 tbsp. of fish sauce
- 1-inch ginger, sliced

Instructions
- Sauté onion in hot oil for 3 minutes.
- Add ginger, water & fish sauce. Boil for 5 minutes, turn the heat to low.
- Add vegetables, cook for 5 minutes.
- Add seafood & let it cook until done. Strain & serve.

Nutrition: Kcal 54 | Protein 2 g | Fiber 0 g | Carbs 7 g | Fat 2.2 g

34. Thai fish soup

(Prep time: 15 minutes | Cook time: 40 minutes |Servings: 4)

Ingredients
- 4 scallions, sliced
- 1" piece of ginger, sliced
- 1 lemongrass
- 2 minced garlic cloves
- 2 tbsp. of oil
- 17 oz. of cod fillet, cut into pieces
- 26 oz. of fish stock
- 1tbsp. of coriander, chopped
- 1 lime's juice
- 2 tbsp. of light soy sauce
- 1 shallot, sliced
- 1 tbsp. of caster sugar
- 2 tbsp. of fish sauce
- Salt & black pepper

Instructions
- Sauté the shallots & scallion in hot oil for 2-3 minutes.
- Add garlic, lemon grass & ginger for 2-3 minutes.
- Add the rest of the ingredients cook for 5-7 minutes.
- Strain & serve.

Nutrition: Kcal 63 | Protein 5 g | Fiber 2 g | Carbs 6 g | Fat 4 g

35. Chinese Fish Soup

(Prep time: 15 minutes | Cook time: 40 minutes |Servings: 8)

Ingredients
- 1 lb. of fish
- Potato starch, as needed
- 1 lb. of pickled mustard greens
- 1 lb. of taro

- 12 cups of water
- 1 fish head
- 5 slices of ginger
- 1 tbsp. of chicken powder
- 8 scallions (white part)
- Salt & sugar, to taste

Instructions

- Coat the fish chunks in potato starch. Fry until golden.
- Do the same with taro.
- In a pan, sauté vegetables in oil until tender.
- Add the rest of the ingredients. Simmer for half an hour.
- Adjust seasoning, strain & serve.

Nutrition: Kcal 55| Protein 2 g | Fiber 1 g | Carbs 7 g | Fat 2 g

36. Ginger Fish Soup

(Prep time: 15 minutes | Cook time: 20 minutes |Servings: 4)

Ingredients

- 1 Tbsp. of cooking oil
- 2" piece of ginger, grated
- 6 cups of chicken stock
- 2 lb. of sole fillets
- 4 Roma tomatoes, diced without seeds
- 2 cups of diced celery
- 1 tsp. + 2 tbsp. of fish sauce
- 2 tsp. of sugar
- 5 shallots, chopped
- 2 cloves of garlic, chopped
- 1 tbsp. of cornstarch

Instructions

- Toss the fish fillets with fish sauce (1 tsp.) & cornstarch.
- Sauté the shallots, ginger & garlic for 2 to 3 minutes in hot oil. Add stock, celery & boil.

- Simmer for 15 minutes. Add fish & tomatoes, cook until done.
- Strain & adjust seasoning, serve.

Nutrition: Kcal 65 | Protein 2 g | Fiber 0 g | Carbs 6 g | Fat 2 g

37. Healthy Jell-O

(Prep time: 15 minutes | Cook time: 20 minutes |Servings: 8)

Ingredients

- 2 Tbsp. beef gelatin, unflavored
- 2 tbsp. of honey
- 4 cups of clear apple juice

Instructions

- Add gelatin to half to ¾ cup of the juice. Whisk well & let it rest for 3 to 5 minutes.
- Add the rest of the juice to a pan simmer on medium heat. Turn the heat off
- Add honey & gelatin mixture. Mix & pour into the dish.
- Keep in the fridge for 4 hours. Slice & serve.

Nutrition: Kcal 44 | Protein 0.1 g | Fiber 1 g | Carbs 15 g | Fat 0 g

38. Finger Jell-O

(Prep time: 15 minutes | Cook time: 5 minutes |Servings: 36)

Ingredients

- 3 Jell-O small boxes
- 4 1/2 cups of boiling water
- 4 envelopes of unflavored gelatin

Instructions

- Boil some water.
- Mix the gelatin with Jell-O. Add the boiling water & stir for 2 to 3 minutes.
- Mix & pour into the dish.
- Keep in the fridge for 4 hours. Slice & serve.

Nutrition: Kcal 84 | Protein 0.1 g | Fiber 1 g | Carbs 15 g | Fat 0 g

40. Jell-O Jugglers

(Prep time: 15 minutes | Cook time: 20 minutes |Servings: 32)

Ingredients
- 4 cups of clear juice
- 4 packets of gelatin

Instructions

- Add gelatin to one cup of cold juice & let it rest for a few minutes.
- Simmer the 3 cups of juice & pour on the gelatin mixture stir until dissolved.
- Pour in a pan. Set in the fridge & serve.

Nutrition: Kcal 44 | Protein 0 g | Fiber 0 g | Carbs 0 g | Fat 0.2 g

Chapter 5: LOW RESIDUE DIET RECIPES

5.1 BREAKFAST

1. Strawberry Spread

(Prep time: 15 minutes | Cook time: 25 minutes |Servings: 1 cup)

Ingredients
- 1 tbsp. of lemon juice
- 2 cups of strawberries
- 1/4 cup of sugar

Instructions
- In a pan, add berries with the rest of the ingredients.
- Place on high flame until it boils; turn the heat low while keep stirring for 15 minutes.
- Cook until the liquid is absorbed. Cool & add to a jar.

Nutrition: Kcal 18 | Protein 0 g | Fiber 1 g | Carbs 5 g | Fat 4 g

2. Apple Cider Sausage

(Prep time: 15 minutes | Cook time: 25 minutes |Servings: 8)

Ingredients
- 1 peeled red apple (cut into wedges)
- 1.7 oz. of chopped yellow squash
- 1 tsp. of garlic powder
- 1 ½ cups of dry cider
- ¼ cup of cream
- 8 chicken sausages
- 1 tbsp. of dried Italian herbs
- 1 tbsp. of olive oil
- ¾ cup of chicken stock
- 2 carrots, peeled

- 1 tbsp. of arrowroot flour

Instructions
- Sauté the sausage in a splash of hot oil until golden brown; take them out on a plate.
- Add the carrots & apple squash to the same pan cook until tender.
- Add garlic powder, cider, herbs & stock. Stir & add flour cook until it thickens.
- Add sausages & cook for 5 to 10 minutes.
- Add cream & simmer for 5-10 minutes more.

Nutrition: Kcal 125 | Protein 9 g | Fiber 3 g | Carbs 12 g | Fat 0.2 g

3. Apple & Pear Pita Pockets

(Prep time: 15 minutes | Cook time: 0 minutes | Servings: 1)

Ingredients

- 1 pita bread
- ½ pear, peeled & chopped
- ½ apple, peeled & chopped
- 1/4 Cup of cottage cheese

Instructions

- In a bowl, mix cheese, apple & pear.
- Cut the pita bread in half but not all the way through.
- Stuff with apple/pear mixture. Drizzle with honey & serve.

Nutrition: Kcal 109 | Protein 1 g | Fiber 1.2 g | Carbs 18 g | Fat 2 g

4. Guacamole Deviled Eggs

(Prep time: 15 minutes | Cook time: 0 minutes | Servings: 6-8)

Ingredients

- 1 avocado, peeled
- 1 tsp. of minced garlic
- 1 tbsp. of lime juice
- 6 eggs, hard-boiled & peeled, halved
- Smoked Paprika, to taste
- 1/4 tsp. of each onion powder & salt
- 2 tsp. of Cilantro

Instructions

- In a bowl, add the egg yolks with the rest of the ingredients.
- Mash it well. Spoon onto the egg white's halves
- Serve.

Nutrition: Kcal 66 | Protein 4 g | Fiber 1 g | Carbs 2 g | Fat 5 g

5. Apple Raisin Pancakes

(Prep time: 15 minutes | Cook time: 10 minutes | Servings: 2)

Ingredients

- 2 tsp. of vanilla
- 1 Cup of unsweetened applesauce
- 2 tsp. of baking powder
- 1 tsp. of cinnamon
- 2 eggs
- 2 tsp. of brown sugar
- 1 & 1/2 Cups of white flour

Instructions

- In a bowl, add eggs & whisk till fluffy.
- Add the rest of the ingredients & fold the mixture.
- Oil spray a pan, pour ¼ cup of the batter on the hot pan.
- Cook on both sides until golden brown. Serve.

Nutrition: Kcal 88 | Protein 2 g | Fiber 1.6 g | Carbs 12 g | Fat 2 g

6. Herbed Avocado Egg Salad

(Prep time: 15 minutes | Cook time: 0 minutes | Servings: 6)

Ingredients

- 1 avocado
- 1 tbsp. of each chopped dill & chopped chives
- ½ cup of Greek yogurt
- 10 hard-boiled eggs, peeled
- 1 lemon's juice
- ½ tsp. of Dijon mustard
- Salt & pepper, to taste
- 1 tbsp. of olive oil

Instructions

- In a bowl, mash the eggs with avocado, do not make it smooth.
- Add the rest of the ingredients. Mix until combined.
- Keep in the fridge for a few hours before serving.

Nutrition: Kcal 230 | Protein 13 g | Fiber 2 g | Carbs 18.7 g | Fat 5 g

7. Tomato Tuna Salad with eggs

(Prep time: 15 minutes | Servings: 3-5)

Ingredients

- 5 tsp. of vinegar
- 1 tbsp. of fresh basil, sliced
- 1 tbsp. of sun-dried tomatoes with 1 tbsp. of oil
- 3 hard-boiled eggs
- 1/8 tsp. of salt
- 5 oz. of tuna, drained

Instructions

- Cut the eggs in half lengthwise.
- Take the egg yolk in a bowl with the rest of the ingredients.
- Mix well & spoon onto the egg whites' halves.
- Serve.

Nutrition: Kcal 87| Protein 1 g | Fiber 1 g | Carbs 11 g | Fat 3 g

8. Apricot Honey Oatmeal

(Prep time: 15 minutes / Servings: 2)

Ingredients

- 1/4 tsp. of cinnamon
- 1/4 Cup of peeled & chopped apricots
- 1 Cup of water
- ½ cup of rolled oats
- 1 tbsp. of honey

Instructions

- Add all ingredients to a bowl & microwave for 2 minutes.
- Mix well & serve.

Nutrition: Kcal 86 | Protein 1 g | Fiber 3 g | Carbs 9 g | Fat 2.2 g

9. High Protein Power Eggs

(Prep time: 15 minutes | Cook time: 12 minutes|Servings: 5)

Ingredients

- ½ red onion, chopped
- 1 cup of yellow squash, cut into cubes
- Garlic salt & black pepper, to taste
- ½ cup of blueberries
- 4 mini sweet peppers
- 4 large eggs

Instructions

- Chop all the vegetables in small sizes.
- Oil spray a pan & place on medium flame. Sauté the vegetables for 5 to 7 minutes.
- Add blueberries cook for 1 minute. Add the whisked eggs.
- Keep whisking & cook to scramble.
- Serve with white bread.

Nutrition: Kcal 379 | Protein 21 g | Fiber 6 g | Carbs 23 g | Fat 18 g

10. Egg Salad

(Prep time: 15 minutes | Cook time: 12 minutes|Servings: 5)

Ingredients

- ¼ cup of mayonnaise
- ⅛ tsp. of paprika
- 1 tsp. of Dijon mustard
- 4 eggs, hard-boiled & chopped
- Salt and pepper, to taste
- 2 tbsp. of diced red bell pepper
- 1 Tbsp. of minced chives

Instructions

- In a bowl, add all ingredients mix until combined.
- Season with salt & pepper.
- Keep in the fridge for a few hours before serving.

Nutrition: Kcal 339 | Protein 13 g | Fiber 0.6 g | Carbs 2.1 g | Fat 30 g

11. Spinach Scrambled Eggs

(Prep time: 15 minutes | Cook time: 5 minutes|Servings: 2)

Ingredients

- 6 eggs
- ½ cup of spinach leaves, chopped
- 3 tbsp. of skim milk
- 1/8 tsp. of each salt & pepper

Instructions

- Oil spray a pan & place on a medium flame.
- Whisk eggs in a bowl with milk, salt & pepper.
- Add eggs to the pan & add spinach. Cook until eggs are done & spinach wilts.
- Serve.

Nutrition: Kcal 233 | Protein 21 g | Fiber 1.2 g | Carbs 4 g | Fat 14 g

12. Asparagus & Bean Frittata

(Prep time: 15 minutes | Cook time: 15minutes|Servings: 4)

Ingredients

- 1 Cup of diced onion
- 2 tbsp. of olive oil
- 1 minced garlic clove
- 14 oz. of canned beans, rinsed
- 1/4 Cup of Parmesan cheese
- 1 Cup of chopped red pepper
- 1 Cup of cooked asparagus, chopped
- 4 eggs
- ½ tsp. of salt

Instructions

- Let the oven preheat to 350°F.
- Heat one tbsp. of oil on medium flame. Sauté the vegetables & beans for 10 minutes.
- Whisk eggs with salt & pepper.
- Add the rest of the oil with eggs. Cook for 10 to 15 minutes on low.
- Add cheese on top, broil for 3 minutes. Slice & serve.

Nutrition: Kcal 167 | Protein 2 g | Fiber 2 g | Carbs 9.8 g | Fat 4.2 g

13. Vegetable Frittata

(Prep time: 15 minutes | Cook time: 45 minutes|Servings: 10)

Ingredients

- 3 bell peppers, diced
- 12 eggs
- 1 peeled zucchini, chopped
- 2 cloves of minced garlic
- 1 red onion, diced
- 1/4 cup of sliced green onion
- 1 tbsp. of oil
- salt & black pepper
- 1/4 cup of skim milk
- 2 oz. of goat cheese

Instructions

- Let the oven preheat to 425°F.
- Oil spray a 9 by 13" pan.
- Toss the zucchini, onion, garlic & peppers with oil, salt & pepper.
- Spread on a baking sheet. Roast for half an hour, stirring halfway through.
- Take the vegetables out & cool for a few minutes.
- Change the oven's temperature to 350°F.
- Whisk eggs with salt, pepper & milk. Add vegetables & mix well.
- Pour in the pan, add goat cheese on top.
- Bake for half an hour & serve.

Nutrition: Kcal 210| Protein 14 g | Fiber 2 g | Carbs 8 g | Fat 13 g

14. Carrot, Clementine & Pineapple Juice

(Prep time: 15 minutes | Cook time: 0minutes|Servings: 3-4)

Ingredients

- 1" piece of peeled ginger
- 1 peeled carrot
- 2 peeled clementine
- ½ of a small pineapple
- Water, as needed

Instructions

- Add all ingredients to a blender.
- Pulse until smooth & strain well.
- Serve.

Nutrition: Kcal 56 | Protein 0.1 g | Fiber 4 g | Carbs 3 g | Fat 1 g

15. Carrot, Pineapple & Ginger Juice

(Prep time: 15 minutes | Cook time: 0minutes|Servings: 3)

Ingredients

- 1 cup of pineapple
- 1" piece of peeled ginger
- 7 to 9 large carrots
- Water, as needed

Instructions

- Add all ingredients to a blender.
- Pulse until smooth & strain well.
- Serve.

Nutrition: Kcal 69 | Protein 2.7 g | Fiber 2 g | Carbs 12 g | Fat 1 g

16. Lychee & Dill Juice

(Prep time: 15 minutes | Cook time: 0minutes|Servings: 2)

Ingredients

- 4 to 5 ice cubes
- 1 lime's juice
- 8.8 oz. of lychees, peeled & deseeded
- 1-2 sprigs of dill

Instructions

- In a blender, add all ingredients with some water.
- Strain & serve.

Nutrition: Kcal 66 | Protein 1 g | Fiber 2 g | Carbs 11 g | Fat 1.2 g

17. Celery Juice

(Prep time: 15 minutes | Cook time: 0minutes|Servings: 2)

Ingredients

- 1 green apple, peeled
- 1 tsp. of lemon juice
- 8 stalks of large celery
- ½ cup of water

Instructions

- Add all ingredients to a blender. Pulse until smooth.
- Strain well & serve.

Nutrition: Kcal 62 | Protein 1.6 g | Fiber 7.2 g | Carbs 12.9 g | Fat 0.6 g

18. Lemon Ginger Turmeric Drink

(Prep time: 15 minutes | Cook time: 0minutes|Servings: 2)

Ingredients

- 2 small lemons' juice
- 1/4 cup fresh ginger, peeled & chopped
- 1/4 tsp. of olive oil
- 1 small orange's juice
- 1/4 cup of fresh turmeric, peeled & chopped
- 1/8 tsp. of black pepper

Instructions

- Add all ingredients to a blender.
- Pulse until smooth, strain & serve in shots glass.

Nutrition: Kcal 78 | Protein 2.8 g | Fiber 0 g | Carbs 11 g | Fat 0.9 g

19. Banana Muffins

(Prep time: 15 minutes | Cook time: 20minutes|Servings: 12)

Ingredients

- 2/3 Cups of skim milk
- 4 eggs
- 1 Cup of white flour
- 1/4 Cup of canola oil
- 1 1/2 Cup of cereal
- 1 Cup of mashed ripe banana
- ½ tsp. of salt
- ½ cup of brown sugar
- 2 tsp. of baking powder

Instructions

- Let the oven preheat to 400°F.
- Add milk & cereal to a bowl, mix & let it rest. Add bananas, oil, eggs & sugar, mix well.
- In a bowl, add salt, flour & baking powder. Mix & add to the wet ingredients.
- Add to the oil sprayed muffin tray. Bake for 15 to 18 minutes.
- Serve.

Nutrition: Kcal 65 | Protein 4 g | Fiber 3 g | Carbs 18.9 g | Fat 4 g

20. Açai Breakfast Bowl

(Prep time: 15 minutes | Cook time: 0minutes|Servings: 2)

Ingredients

- 1 oz. of cornflakes
- 2 oz. of frozen raspberries
- 2 tbsp. of maple syrup
- 2 oz. of instant oats
- A pinch of salt
- 1 ½ cups of almond milk
- 1 tbsp. of acai powder
- 1 tsp. of mixed spice

Instructions

- Heat the milk on a low flame.
- Add the oats & keep mixing.

- Add acai powder, raspberries, maple syrup & mixed spice. Cook for 3 to 4 minutes.
- Turn the heat off.
- Let it rest for 2 to 3 minutes. Add the crunchy flakes & serve.

Nutrition: Kcal 105 | Protein 3 g | Fiber 3 g | Carbs 11 g | Fat 1.2 g

21. Very Berry Khatta

(Prep time: 15 minutes | Cook time: 0minutes|Servings: 1)

Ingredients

- 1 orange wedge
- ¼ cup of grape juice
- Crushed ice, as needed
- 4 mulberries
- 2 lime slices
- 2 tbsp. of kala khatta syrup
- Black salt, as needed

Instructions

- Crush 2 mulberries with orange & half of the lime.
- Add the rest of the ingredients. Adjust seasoning.
- Serve.

Nutrition: Kcal 55 | Protein 0 g | Fiber 1 g | Carbs 3 g | Fat 0 g.

22. Apple Blueberry Friends

(Prep time: 15 minutes | Cook time: 20minutes|Servings: 12)

Ingredients

- ½ cup + ¼ cup of white flour (self-rising)
- Puree of 2 peeled red apples
- Half cup of blueberries
- 1/3 cup of skim milk
- 2 oz. of almond meal
- 1/4 cup of grapeseed oil

- 5 egg whites
- 3 tbsp. of stevia powder
- 1 tsp. of vanilla essence

Instructions

- Let the oven preheat to 390 F.
- Add vanilla essence, flours, stevia & almond meal. Mix.
- Add oil, milk, blueberries & apple, mix well.
- Whisk the egg whites till soft peaks form & add the rest of the mixture; fold.
- Add to the prepared pan & bake for 20 to 30 minutes at 356°F.
- Let it sit for 5 minutes before taking it out of the mold.

Nutrition: Kcal 89 | Protein 0 g | Fiber 1.2 g | Carbs 12 g | Fat 2 g

23. Seedless Raspberry Sauce

(Prep time: 15 minutes | Cook time: 20minutes|Servings: 2)

Ingredients

- 1/4 cup of sugar
- 1 tsp. of lemon juice
- 1 ½ cups of raspberries

Instructions

- In a pan, add all ingredients & stir, let it come to a boil.
- Cool for a few minutes, pass through a fine sieve. Keep mashing & you will get the sauce.
- Store in a jar.

Nutrition: Kcal 37| Protein 0 g | Fiber 0 g | Carbs 9 g | Fat 0.2 g

24. Aloo Masala

(Prep time: 15 minutes | Cook time: 20minutes|Servings: 2)

Ingredients

- 17.6 oz. peeled potato, cut into chunks
- 1/4 cup of smooth cashew butter
- 2 tbsp. of raisins
- 1 tsp. of powdered garlic
- 4 peeled carrots, cut into chunks
- 2 tsp. of garam masala
- ½ cup of coriander leaves
- 1 tsp. of ground cumin
- 3.5 oz. of baby spinach
- 1 tbsp. of brown sugar
- 1 cup of vegetable stock
- Salt and black pepper, to taste
- 1 lemon, sliced into wedges

Instructions

- Sauté garlic & onion in hot oil for 1 minute.
- Add cumin, vegetables, salt, pepper & garam masala, cook for 2 to 3 minutes.
- Add raisins, stock & sugar; cook for 10-12 minutes.
- Add spinach, coriander & nut butter. Cook for 2-3 minutes.
- Serve with lemon wedges.

Nutrition: Kcal 156 | Protein 0.1 g | Fiber 3 g | Carbs 189 g | Fat 12g

25. Boost Detox Juice

(Prep time: 15 minutes | Cook time: 20minutes|Servings: 2)

Ingredients

- 1 orange
- 1 green apple peeled & cored
- 1/4 tsp. of chopped ginger
- 3 kale leaves
- 1 carrot, chopped
- 1 cup of baby spinach
- ½ peeled lemon
- 2 cups of water

Instructions

- Add all ingredients to a blender. Pulse until smooth.
- Strain well & serve.

Nutrition: Kcal 116 | Protein 3 g | Fiber 4 g | Carbs 17 g | Fat 0.2 g

5.2 LUNCH

1. Chicken Vegetable Pasta Soup

(Prep time: 15 minutes | Cook time: 20minutes|Servings: 4)

Ingredients

- 1 potato, chopped
- 5 cups of chicken broth
- ½ cup of cooked small pasta
- 1 carrot, chopped
- ½ cup of tomato flesh with no skin/seeds
- 1 bunch of asparagus tips

Instructions

- In a pan, add potatoes, carrot & broth. Let it come to a boil, turn the heat low & cook until tender.
- Add asparagus tips & tomatoes, cook until tender.
- Add cooked pasta, heat it through & serve.

Nutrition: Kcal 116 | Protein 10 g | Fiber 3 g | Carbs 17 g | Fat 2 g

2. Asian Chicken Salad

(Prep time: 15 minutes | Cook time: 0minutes|Servings: 4)

Ingredients

- 1 celery, thinly slice
- 2 tbsp. of lime & ginger dressing
- 1/4 Cup of red bell pepper, sliced without seeds
- 1 carrot, shredded
- ½ cup of chicken breast, sliced into strips
- 1/4 Cup of mangoes

Instructions

- Add all ingredients to a bowl toss well.
- Serve.

Nutrition: Kcal 72 | Protein 7 g | Fiber 4 g | Carbs 8 g | Fat 1.8 g

3. Basil Zoodle Frittata

(Prep time: 15 minutes | Cook time: 35minutes|Servings: 4)

Ingredients

- 1 tsp. of powdered garlic
- ½ cup of cottage cheese
- 1/4 cup of sliced fine chives
- ½ cup of bread crumbs
- 2 zucchinis, spiralized
- 6 eggs
- 1/4 cup of torn basil leaves
- Salt, a pinch

- 1 tbsp. of olive oil

Instructions

- Let the oven preheat to 350°F.
- In the pie dish, press the crumbs into a base
- Bake for 10 minutes, press down once more.
- Boil the zucchini, sprinkle some salt & drain. Add to a bowl with the rest of the ingredients.
- Mix well & place on the baked pie crust.
- Bake for 20 to 30 minutes. Slice & serve.

Nutrition: Kcal 102 | Protein 2 g | Fiber 3 g | Carbs 18 g | Fat 4 g

4. Ciabatta Pizza

(Prep time: 15 minutes | Cook time: 20minutes|Servings: 4)

Ingredients

- 2 cups of tomato sauce
- 2 cups of mozzarella cheese
- 1 small zucchini, cut into ¼" rounds
- 1-pound loaf of ciabatta
- ½ cup of sliced mushrooms
- 2 tbsp. of basil

Instructions

- Let the oven preheat to 400°F.
- Slice the bread loaf lengthwise & take some of the bread out from inside.
- Place on a baking sheet. Add sauce on top & spread.
- Add zucchini & mushrooms on top, end with cheese & basil.
- Bake for 12-15 minutes.

Nutrition: Kcal 263| Protein 13g | Fiber 2 g | Carbs 36.5 g | Fat 8 g

5. Low Fiber Beet Carrot Soup

(Prep time: 15 minutes | Cook time: 0minutes|Servings: 4)

Ingredients

- 4 cups of vegetable broth
- Salt, to taste
- 1 carrot, sliced
- 1 can of cooked beets (simple, not pickled)

Instructions

- In a pan, add broth & carrots.
- Boil & simmer until tender.
- Add beets & cook for a few minutes. Pulse with a stick blender.
- Adjust seasoning & serve.

Nutrition: Kcal 90| Protein 2 g | Fiber 3.1 g | Carbs 22 g | Fat 1 g

6. Broth Braised Asparagus Tips

(Prep time: 5 minutes | Cook time: 5minutes|Servings: 2)

Ingredients

- 1 tbsp. of olive oil
- 1 cup of asparagus tips
- ½ cup of chicken broth
- One slice of lemon peel

Instructions

- Boil the broth with oil.
- Add the rest of the ingredients. Cook for 3 to 4 minutes.
- Serve.

Nutrition: Kcal 44 | Protein 0.1 g | Fiber 1 g | Carbs 7 g | Fat 0.2 g

7. Lemon Chicken Rice Soup

(Prep time: 15 minutes | Cook time: 20minutes|Servings: 2)

Ingredients

- 2 cups of baby spinach

- 1 carrot, chopped
- 1 cup of cooked & shredded chicken breast
- 1 celery stalk, chopped
- 4 cups of chicken broth
- 3 eggs
- 1/4 cup of sushi rice
- 1 lemon's juice

Instructions

- In an instant pot, add rice, carrots, broth & celery. Cook for 10 minutes on high pressure.
- Release for 15 minutes. Select sauté & add chicken.
- Cook for a few minutes. Add whisked eggs slowly, add lemon juice & spinach.
- Cook for a few minutes. Serve.

Nutrition: Kcal 163 | Protein 11 g | Fiber 1.2 g | Carbs 20 g | Fat 5 g

8. Bean and Couscous Salad

(Prep time: 15 minutes | Cook time: 0minutes|Servings: 4)

Ingredients

- 1 ½ Cup of boiling water
- 2 Cups of tomatoes, peeled, chopped without seeds
- 1 Cup of chopped bell peppers, without seeds
- 1 Cup of couscous
- 2 Cups of cooked black beans
- 1/4 tsp. of pepper
- 1 onion, chopped
- 2 minced garlic cloves
- ½ tsp. of salt
- ½ cup of rice vinegar
- 1/4 Cup of olive oil

Instructions

- Add water & couscous. Let it rest, covered, until all liquid is absorbed.
- Add the rest of the ingredients, mix & adjust seasoning.
- Serve.

Nutrition: Kcal 132 | Protein 4 g | Fiber 5 g | Carbs 17 g | Fat 2 g

9. Apple Sausage Pasta

(Prep time: 15 minutes | Cook time: 25minutes|Servings: 4)

Ingredients

- 1 peeled Green apple, chopped
- 14 oz. of passata
- 1 onion, diced
- 1 cup of shredded cheddar cheese
- 16 oz. of chicken sausages
- 2 tsp. of garlic powder
- 1 tbsp. of olive oil
- 17 oz. of chicken stock
- 10 oz. of pasta
- Salt & pepper, to taste

Instructions

- Heat the oil & sauté garlic, sausage, onion for 10 minutes.
- Cool & slice the sausages thinly, add to the pan with apples.
- Cook until the apple is tender.
- Add passata & stock; mix well. Add salt & pepper, boil.
- Add pasta, cook, until done. Add cheese before serving.

Nutrition: Kcal 176 | Protein 4 g | Fiber 3 g | Carbs 21 g | Fat 5 g

10. Egg Potato Bites

(Prep time: 15 minutes | Cook time: 25minutes|Servings: 12)

Ingredients

- 8 oz. of cooked & peeled potato, chopped
- 1 cup of cottage cheese, pureed
- 8 eggs
- Salt, to taste
- 2 oz. of Swiss cheese

Instructions

- Let the oven preheat to 325°F. Oil spray a 12 cup muffin tin.
- In a bowl, mix the cottage cheese, potatoes, salt & egg. Add to the cups, sprinkle with cheese on top.
- Bake for half an hour.

Nutrition: Kcal 90| Protein 8 g | Fiber 1 g | Carbs 3 g | Fat 4 g

11. Greek Yogurt Fettuccini Alfredo

(Prep time: 15 minutes | Cook time: 10minutes|Servings: 4)

Ingredients

- 1 ½ cups of yogurt
- ½ cup of grated parmesan
- ¼ cup of fresh parsley
- 1 pound of fettuccini
- 1 tsp. of black pepper
- 3 tbsp. of minced garlic

Instructions

- Cook pasta as per package instructions, drain all but one cup of water.
- Add the rest of the ingredients to a bowl, add pasta water as needed.
- Whisk well and add to the pasta.
- Heat it through. Serve.

Nutrition: Kcal 170 | Protein 8 g | Fiber 1 g | Carbs 20 g | Fat 6 g

12. Brown Rice Greek Salad

(Prep time: 15 minutes | Cook time: 0minutes|Servings: 4)

Ingredients

- ½ cup of canned white beans, rinsed
- 1/4 Cup of avocado, diced
- ½ cup of fresh spinach
- ½ cup of Brown rice, cooked
- 1 tsp. of red wine vinegar
- 2 tbsp. of Feta cheese, crumbled
- ½ cup of tomatoes, no seeds
- ½ cup of English Cucumber, no seeds
- 1 tbsp. of red onion, chopped
- 2 tbsp. of olive oil
- Salt and pepper, to taste

Instructions

- Add all ingredients to a bowl. Toss & adjust seasoning.
- Serve.

Nutrition: Kcal 72 | Protein 0.1 g | Fiber 1.2 g | Carbs 18.7 g | Fat 2 g

13. Avocado Smash Chips

(Prep time: 15 minutes | Cook time: 30minutes|Servings: 5)

Ingredients

- 1 slice of honey soy tofu, cubed
- 3.5 oz. of cream cheese
- 2 peeled sweet potatoes
- Salt & pepper, to taste
- 1/4 cup of coriander, chopped
- 1 tsp. of sumac
- 1 avocado
- 1/4 cup of lime juice

Instructions

- Let the oven preheat to 400°F.
- Oil spray 2 baking sheets.
- Cut the sweet potatoes into thin slices. Place on the prepared tray.
- Spray the slices & bake for 20 minutes.
- Flip & bake for 10 minutes after oil spraying them.

- In a bowl, smash the avocado with salt, coriander, lime juice, sumac & pepper.
- Serve the potato chips with avocado mix & cube of tofu on top.

Nutrition: Kcal 45 | Protein 3 g | Fiber 2 g | Carbs 14 g | Fat 3 g

14. Citrus Swordfish

(Prep time: 15 minutes | Cook time: 0minutes|Servings: 2)

Ingredients
- 1 tbsp. of fresh thyme, chopped
- 2 tbsp. of mix Lemon, lime & orange lime zest
- 2 swordfish steaks (6 oz. each)
- 1 tbsp. of fresh parsley, chopped
- 1 tbsp. of olive oil

Instructions
- Heat the broiler.
- Mix the oil with herbs. Rub on the fish.
- Broil for 3-4 minutes, flip & broil until done.
- Serve with zest mixture on top.

Nutrition: Kcal 232| Protein 34 g | Fiber 1 g | Carbs 3 g | Fat 9 g

15. Vanilla Soy Pudding

(Prep time: 5 minutes | Cook time: 5minutes|Servings: 4)

Ingredients
- 1/4 cup of cold water
- ½ tsp. of vanilla
- 1 1/4 cup of vanilla soy milk
- 1/4 oz. of unflavored gelatin
- 1 cup of tofu

Instructions
- Mix the gelatin with water & stir. Let it rest for 10 minutes.

- Heat the milk adds to a blender with the rest of the ingredients.
- Pulse until smooth. Pour in a container keep it in the fridge for 2 hours.
- Serve.

Nutrition: Kcal 105 | Protein 9 g | Fiber 1.2 g | Carbs 5 g | Fat 5 g

16. Chicken Pasta Salad

(Prep time: 10 minutes | Cook time: 15minutes|Servings: 4)

Ingredients
- 1 Cup of cooked & cubed chicken
- 1 tsp. of Italian seasoning
- ½ cup of peas
- ½ pound of pasta
- ½ cup of Ranch dressing
- 1 tbsp. of Parmesan cheese, grated

Instructions
- Cook pasta as per package instructions
- Drain & add to a bowl with the rest of the ingredients.
- Toss well & serve.

Nutrition: Kcal 145 | Protein 12 g | Fiber 1 g | Carbs 13 g | Fat 5 g

17. Veggie Stir Fry

(Prep time: 10 minutes | Cook time: 15minutes|Servings: 4)

Ingredients
- 1 tbsp. of chopped chives
- 1 cup of julienned carrots
- 2 tbsp. of sesame oil
- 1 cup of green beans
- 1 cup of julienned zucchini
- 1/4 cup of coriander, chopped
- 1 peeled & sliced red apple
- 1 tbsp. of grated ginger

Instructions

- In a pan, add oil & heat.
- Sauté the ginger & chives. Add the rest of the ingredients cook until tender-crisp.
- Serve with white rice.

Nutrition: Kcal 87| Protein 3 g | Fiber 3 g | Carbs 13 g | Fat 3 g

18. Honey-Herb Chicken

(Prep time: 10 minutes | Cook time: 10minutes|Servings: 4)

Ingredients

- 4 chicken breast halves (boneless & skinless)
- 1 tbsp. of honey
- 2 tbsp. of lime juice
- 1-2 tbsp. of coriander

Instructions

- Pound the chicken into half" of thickness.
- Mix the rest of the ingredients & brush the chicken with it.
- Oil spray the grill & grill for 5 minutes on one side.
- Slice & serve.

Nutrition: Kcal 149 | Protein 27 g | Fiber 1 g | Carbs 5 g | Fat 1.5 g

19. Pasta Bake

(Prep time: 10 minutes | Cook time: 45minutes|Servings: 4)

Ingredients

- 7 oz. of canned asparagus, sliced
- 1 tsp. of mixed herbs
- 14 oz. of pasta
- 2 cups of chicken stock
- 2 oz. of white bread crumbs
- 18 oz. of peeled pumpkin, cut into chunks
- 2 tbsp. of oil
- 5 oz. of grated cheese

Instructions

- Let the oven preheat to 420°F.
- Toss the pumpkin with 1 tbsp. of oil & roast until golden & tender.
- Cook the pasta until done.
- In a bowl, add olive oil & breadcrumbs; stock mix well.
- Add the rest of the ingredients. Mix.
- Add to the baking dish bake for half an hour. Serve.

Nutrition: Kcal 145 | Protein 3 g | Fiber 5 g | Carbs 18.7 g | Fat 6 g

20. Chicken Parmesan

(Prep time: 10 minutes | Cook time: 45minutes|Servings: 4)

Ingredients

- 4 chicken legs
- Breadcrumbs, as needed
- ¼ cup of water
- 2 tbsp. of oil
- 1 egg
- 4 slices of cheese
- 1 can of (15 oz.) chopped tomatoes
- ½ tsp. of mix oregano, thyme & basil
- Salt & pepper

Instructions

- Whisk egg with 1 tbsp. of water.
- Coat the chicken in egg mixture then in breadcrumbs.
- Oil spray them generously & bake until cooked at 400°F.
- Add the rest of the ingredients in a bowl (except for cheese), mix & pour over chicken. Transfer to a pan.
- Cook for 15-20 minutes more on medium flame.

- Place cheese on top cook until it melts.

Nutrition: Kcal 176 | Protein 12.2 g | Fiber 3 g | Carbs 17.7 g | Fat 7 g

21. Sweet Potato Soup

(Prep time: 10 minutes | Cook time: 35minutes|Servings: 4)

Ingredients

- 2 tbsp. of olive oil
- ½ cup of white onion, diced
- 2 tbsp. of all-purpose flour
- 3 cups of sweet potatoes, peeled & cubed
- 3 cups of chicken broth
- Salt, to taste
- ⅛ tsp. of ground cloves
- 2 tbsp. of brown sugar
- ½ tsp. of ground turmeric
- 2 cups of soy milk
- ¼ tsp. of ground cinnamon

Instructions

- Boil the sweet potatoes until tender. Drain.
- In a pan, mix the oil & flour cook until it turns caramel color. Add sugar & broth.
- Boil & simmer, add the rest of the ingredients. Cook for 5 minutes.
- Turn the heat off & blend with a stick blender.
- Cook for 5 to 10 minutes. Adjust seasoning & serve.

Nutrition: Kcal 366| Protein 17.1 g | Fiber 1 g | Carbs 43.6 g | Fat 13.7 g

22. Green Bean Potato Salad

(Prep time: 10 minutes | Cook time: 10minutes|Servings: 4-6)

Ingredients

- 6 red potatoes, small & peeled, cubed
- 1 small onion, sliced thin
- 1 tsp. of sugar
- 1/3 Cup of olive oil
- 1 tbsp. of garlic powder
- 1/4 Cup of red wine vinegar
- 1 ½ Pound of fresh green beans
- 1/4 Cup of rice vinegar

Instructions

- Boil the green beans & potatoes for 7 minutes, till tender-crisp.
- Drain & add to the cold water. Drain.
- Add onions, beans & potatoes. Add the rest of the ingredients to a bowl, whisk & pour on the salad. Toss & serve.

Nutrition: Kcal 78| Protein 2 g | Fiber 3 g | Carbs 12 g | Fat 3 g

23. Beetroot Tarte Tatin

(Prep time: 10 minutes | Cook time: 35minutes|Servings: 4-6)

Ingredients

- 1 sheet of puff pastry, thawed
- 1 tbsp. of brown sugar
- 8 basil leaves
- 0.5 oz. of butter
- 8 small cooked beetroots, sliced thick
- 1.7 oz. of crumbled feta cheese
- 1 tbsp. of balsamic vinegar

Instructions

- Let the oven preheat to 390 F.
- Oil spray a 9" pan (pie pan).
- Add beetroot, butter, sugar & vinegar to a pan simmer for 15 minutes.
- Cool for a few minutes, add to the pie pan place the pastry sheet on top.
- Bake for 25 minutes. Cool, slice & serve.

Nutrition: Kcal 92 | Protein 4 g | Fiber 3 g | Carbs 13 g | Fat 3 g

24. Herb-Crusted Tilapia

(Prep time: 10 minutes | Cook time: 10minutes|Servings: 2)

Ingredients
- 2 tilapia fillets
- 2 tbsp. of mixed herbs
- 1 tbsp. of flour
- 1 tbsp. of olive oil
- 1 egg whisk with 1 tbsp. of water
- Half cup of panko

Instructions
- With flout coat the fish fillets lightly.
- Mix herbs with panko. Coat the fish in egg, then panko mixture.
- Drizzle some oil in a pan, place fish & cook on a medium flame for 3 minutes on one side. Serve.

Nutrition: Kcal 317 | Protein 39 g | Fiber 1.5 g | Carbs 15 g | Fat 11 g

5.3 DINNER

1. Grilled Salmon Steaks

(Prep time: 10 minutes | Cook time: 10minutes|Servings: 2)

Ingredients

- 1 tsp. of cooking oil
- 2 salmon steaks
- 2 tbsp. of dipping sauce

Instructions

- Heat the grill.
- Brush the fish fillets with sauce grill for 5 minutes on one side.

Nutrition: Kcal 295 | Protein 31 g | Fiber 0 g | Carbs 7 g | Fat 17 g

2. Fiesta Chicken Tacos

(Prep time: 10 minutes | Cook time: 20minutes|Servings: 8)

Ingredients

- 1 tbsp. of olive oil
- ¼ tsp. of salt
- ½ tsp. of ground cumin
- 1 pound of chicken breast, skinless & boneless, cut into thin strips
- 1 cup of each sliced red bell pepper & red onion
- 8 corn tortillas (six inches)
- 1 cup of mixed salad greens

Instructions

- Season chicken with cumin. Sauté in hot oil for 3 minutes.
- Take it out on a plate.
- Sauté the onion & bell pepper in 1 tsp. of oil for 3 minutes.
- Add chicken back in the pan add salt.
- Warm the tortillas & add chicken mixture (1/3 cup) with 2 tbsp. of mixed greens.
- Roll & serve.

Nutrition: Kcal 320| Protein 30.3 g | Fiber 3.8 g | Carbs 36.1 g | Fat 6.4 g

3. Taco Soup

(Prep time: 10 minutes | Cook time: 45minutes|Servings: 8)

Ingredients

- 1 packet of ranch dressing
- 1 small onion
- 3 cups of water
- 1 pound of lean ground beef
- 1 bag of frozen corn
- 15 oz. canned tomato sauce
- 1 packet of taco seasoning

Instructions

- Sauté meat until no longer pink.
- Push to a side & sauté onion until translucent. Drain the fat.
- Add the rest of the ingredients. Simmer on low flame for half an hour.
- Serve.

Nutrition: Kcal 165 | Protein 6.5 g | Fiber 1.9 g | Carbs 18.7 g | Fat 7.5 g

4. Shrimp Scampi Pizza

(Prep time: 10 minutes | Cook time: 20minutes|Servings: 8)

Ingredients

- 1 pack of 13.8 oz. of pizza dough
- 1 pound of peeled shrimp, cooked & sliced
- 1 tbsp. of cornmeal
- 2 cups of shredded mozzarella
- Half cup of ricotta cheese
- 6 cloves of roasted garlic
- 1 tbsp. of dried basil

Instructions

- Let the oven preheat to 400°F.
- Oil spray a baking pan.

- Stretch the dough over cornmeal & place it in the baking pan.
- Bake for 8 minutes.
- Mix ricotta & garlic & spread on the dough. Add shrimps, then mozzarella & basil.
- Bake for 12 minutes. Slice & serve.

Nutrition: Kcal 175| Protein 14 g | Fiber 1 g | Carbs 18.7 g | Fat 5 g

5. Metabolic Soup

(Prep time: 10 minutes | Cook time: 45minutes|Servings: 18)

Ingredients
- 2 quarts of water
- 2 cans of 32oz. stewed tomatoes
- 2 cups of sliced celery
- 2 cups of sliced onions
- 6 cups of bok choy
- 2 cups of sliced bell pepper
- 1 tbsp. of rosemary
- 2 cups of sliced carrots
- 2 chicken thighs
- 1 tbsp. of thyme
- Salt and pepper, to taste

Instructions
- In a pot, add water & chicken, boil for half an hour.
- Take the chicken out & debone it.
- Add all the ingredients to the broth.
- Add more water if necessary, cook until everything is tender and serve.

Nutrition: Kcal 56| Protein 3.1 g | Fiber 1.1 g | Carbs 11.9 g | Fat 0.2 g

6. Detox Soup

(Prep time: 10 minutes | Cook time: 35minutes|Servings: 8)

Ingredients
- 1 yellow onion, diced

- 4 carrots, chopped
- 6 cloves of minced garlic minced
- 2" of ginger peeled & chopped
- 1 tbsp. of olive oil
- 4 celery stalks, chopped
- 1 can of (14 oz.) chickpeas, rinsed
- 1 can of 14 oz. tomatoes
- 8 oz. of mushrooms
- 1 small head of broccoli, broken into florets
- ¼ cup of chopped fresh parsley
- 1 tbsp. of turmeric powder
- 1 tsp. of cinnamon
- 2 cups of spinach
- 1 bay leaf
- salt and pepper to taste
- 8 cups of vegetable
- 1 cup of chopped purple cabbage
- 1 lemon's juice

Instructions
- Sauté the garlic, onion & ginger in hot oil for a few seconds.
- Add mushrooms, celery, tomatoes, carrots & broccoli, cook for 3 minutes
- Add the spices and chickpeas & stock. Let it come to a boil, reduce heat & simmer for 15 minutes.
- Add lemon juice, spinach, parsley & cabbage. Simmer for 5 minutes.
- Serve.

Nutrition: Kcal 89 | Protein 3 g | Fiber 4 g | Carbs 13 g | Fat 4 g

7. Low & Slow Pulled Pork

(Prep time: 20 minutes | Cook time: 5 hours |Servings: 10)

Ingredients
- 1 cup of dark brown sugar
- 1 tbsp. of Creole seasoning
- ½ cup of granulated garlic

- ½ cup of kosher salt
- 5 pounds of pork blade roast
- 1/2cup of paprika
- 2 tbsp. of dried minced onion
- 1 tbsp. of red pepper
- 1 tbsp. of ground cumin
- 1 tbsp. of black pepper
- 1/4 cup of Worcestershire sauce
- 1 minced garlic clove
- 3/4 cup of cider vinegar
- 1 tbsp. of lemon juice
- ½ cup of ketchup
- 1 tbsp. of brown sugar
- ½ tsp. of dry mustard
- 2 tbsp. of onions
- 1 dash of red pepper
- Apple juice, as needed

Instructions

- In a bowl, mix paprika (half cup), Creole seasoning (1 tbsp.), cumin (1 tbsp.), dark brown sugar (1 cup), granulated onion, red pepper, granulated garlic & salt (half cup). Mix & store in a container.
- In a pan, add the rest of the ingredients except for pork. Let it come to a boil, turn the heat low & simmer for 40 minutes. Divide this into 2 containers.
- Season the pork with spice rub generously. Wrap in plastic wrap & keep in the fridge overnight.
- Place the meat at room temperature for 45 minutes before cooking.
- Smoke the meat for 2 hours at 225-250°F.
- Spray the meat with apple juice & place wrap in the aluminum foil.

- Smoke for 2 more hours, smoke until the internal temperature reaches 195° F.
- Cool for half an hour, shred & serve with sauce.

Nutrition: Kcal 134 | Protein 17 g | Fiber 1.2 g | Carbs 11 g | Fat 8 g

8. Zucchini Lasagna

(Prep time: 20 minutes | Cook time: 40 minutes |Servings: 10)

Ingredients

- 1 tsp. of powdered onion
- 1 tsp. of powdered garlic
- Salt & pepper, to taste
- 1 tbsp. of chopped chives
- 9 lasagna sheets
- 1 tbsp. of dried oregano
- 8.8 oz. of ricotta
- 1.7 oz. of shredded cheddar
- 12 oz. of passata
- 28 oz. of grated zucchini

Instructions

- Let the oven preheat to 400°F.
- Sauté the zucchini, onion & garlic powder for 3 minutes in hot oil.
- Add cheddar & ricotta (3/4 tub), salt & pepper.
- Cook the lasagna sheets for 5 to 6 minutes.
- Layer the cooked sheets with zucchini & cheese mix, add chives & oregano on each later, lastly, add a layer of passata.
- Keep doing the layers.
- Add some cheese on top. Bake at 350° F for half an hour.
- Serve.

Nutrition: Kcal 109 | Protein 4 g | Fiber 3 g | Carbs 21 g | Fat 6 g

9. Simple Salmon with Dill Sauce

(Prep time: 10 minutes | Cook time: 40 minutes |Servings: 6)

Ingredients

- 2 tbsp. of soy sauce
- ½ cup of chopped cucumber
- Black pepper, to taste
- 2 pounds of salmon fillet
- ½ cup of sour cream
- Olive oil, to taste
- 1 tsp. of fresh dill

Instructions

- Let the oven preheat to 450°F.
- Pour the soy sauce on the fish & season with salmon. Roast for 10 minutes for each" of thickness,
- Mix the rest of the ingredients & serve with salmon.

Nutrition: Kcal 288 | Protein 31 g | Fiber 0 g | Carbs 5 g | Fat 17 g

10. Portobello Mushroom Pizza

(Prep time: 20 minutes | Cook time: 40 minutes |Servings: 1)

Ingredients

- 1 Portobello Mushroom
- 1 oz. of Mozzarella Cheese
- ½ cup of marinara sauce

Instructions

- Let the oven preheat to 425°F.
- Scrape the mushroom's inside mix the insides with a half cup of sauce.
- Add to the mushroom bowl. Add cheese on top.
- Bake for 20 minutes.

Nutrition: Kcal 133 | Protein 10 g | Fiber 1.2 g | Carbs 11 g | Fat 6 g

11. Tex-Mex Chili

(Prep time: 20 minutes | Cook time: 30 minutes |Servings: 6)

Ingredients

- 2 packets of Taco Seasoning
- 1 can diced tomato with chilies
- 21 oz. of black bean
- 1 pound of lean ground beef & ground turkey
- 22 oz. of pepper & onion blend

Instructions

- Brown the meats & drain all fat.
- Add the rest of the ingredients simmer for 20 minutes. Do not add extra water.
- Serve.

Nutrition: Kcal 176| Protein 18 g | Fiber 1.2 g | Carbs 17 g | Fat 6 g

12. Southeastern Seasoned Catfish

(Prep time: 10 minutes | Cook time: 10 minutes |Servings: 2)

Ingredients

- 2 tsp. of dried minced onion
- 1/4 tsp. of mustard powder
- 2 catfish fillets, boneless & skinless
- ½ tsp. of paprika
- ½ tsp. of garlic powder
- 1/4 tsp. of cayenne pepper

Instructions

- In a bowl, add all ingredients except for fish. Mix and sprinkle on the fish generously.
- Oil spray the butter paper & place the fish on top. Broil for 5 minutes' flip & broil for 3-4 minutes more.
- Serve.

Nutrition: Kcal 239| Protein 27 g | Fiber 1 g | Carbs 0 g | Fat 14 g

13. Winter Apple Poke Bowl

(Prep time: 10 minutes | Cook time: 50 minutes |Servings: 2)

Ingredients

- ½ cup of parsley & coriander
- ½ peeled & chopped butternut pumpkin
- 1 red apple, peeled & sliced
- 1 packet of precooked white rice
- ½ cup of chopped chives
- 2 tbsp. of lemon juice
- 1 tsp. of grated ginger
- 7 oz. of diced halloumi
- 2 tbsp. of olive oil
- 1 tbsp. of honey

Instructions

- Let the oven preheat to 390 F.
- Roast the pumpkin for 30-40 minutes until tender.
- Cook halloumi on a pan until golden.
- In a bowl, add the rest of the ingredients. Top with halloumi & pumpkin. Serve

Nutrition: Kcal 178 | Protein 3 g | Fiber 4 g | Carbs 14 g | Fat 4 g

14. Creamy Tuscan Chicken Pasta

(Prep time: 10 minutes | Cook time: 20 minutes |Servings: 4)

Ingredients

- 1.5 lb. of diced chicken breast, boneless & skinless
- 2 tbsp. of olive oil
- 10 oz. of short pasta
- 3-4 garlic cloves, minced
- 1 tsp. of Italian seasoning
- 2 tbsp. of flour
- Salt and pepper to taste

- ½ cup of Parmesan cheese
- 8 oz. sun-dried (in oil) tomatoes, chopped
- 3 cups of almond milk
- 3 cups of baby spinach

Instructions

- Cook pasta as per package instructions.
- Mix the chicken with salt, pepper, oil, garlic & Italian seasoning.
- Cook chicken in a drizzle of hot oil for 2 to 3 minutes.
- Add the tomatoes & cook for 5 to 7 minutes.
- Whisk flour & milk. Add to the pan cook for 3-4 minutes.
- Add spinach, then add pasta with cheese, stir & serve.

Nutrition: Kcal 368 | Protein 27 g | Fiber 4 g | Carbs 36 g | Fat 13 g

15. French Oven Beef Stew

(Prep time: 10 minutes | Cook time: 5 hours |Servings: 6)

Ingredients

- 1 cup of diced fennel bulb
- 4 potatoes
- 1 celery stalk
- 1 lb. stew beef
- 6 carrots
- 4 parsnips
- 1/4 cup quick-cooking tapioca
- 1 tsp. of ground basil
- 1 Tbsp. of sugar
- ½ tsp. of salt
- 1 cup of tomato juice
- ½ tsp. of black pepper

Instructions

- Let the oven preheat to 300°F.

- Slice the beef into cubes. Peel & chop vegetables.
- In a dish, add all ingredients except for potatoes. Bake for 3 hours.
- Add potatoes & bake for 1 hour more. Serve.

Nutrition: Kcal 213| Protein 30 g | Fiber 2 g | Carbs 16 g | Fat 8g

16. Prawn & Tomato Spaghetti

(Prep time: 10 minutes | Cook time: 20 minutes |Servings: 6)

Ingredients
- 1 tbsp. of olive oil
- 2 tbsp. of chopped parsley leaves
- 4 garlic cloves, sliced
- 6 tomatoes, chopped without seeds
- 13 oz. of spaghetti
- 20 green prawns, peeled & deveined

Instructions
- Cook noodles as per package instructions. Drain all but a half cup of water.
- Sauté garlic in hot oil for 1 minute.
- Add prawns cook for 2 to 3 minutes.
- Add tomatoes & cook for 2 minutes.
- Add parsley & pasta. Toss & serve.

Nutrition: Kcal 490 | Protein 33 g | Fiber 1.2 g | Carbs 50 g | Fat 6.5 g

17. Lemon Pepper Turkey

(Prep time: 10 minutes | Cook time: 20 minutes |Servings: 4)

Ingredients
- 1 tbsp. of lemon pepper seasoning
- 1 tsp. of kosher salt
- 2 minced cloves garlic
- 2 lemons
- ½ cup of all-purpose flour
- 2 tbsp. of butter

- 1 lb. turkey breasts, boneless & skinless halved
- 2 tbsp. olive oil
- ½ cup of Chicken broth

Instructions
- Let the oven preheat to 400°F.
- In a bowl, add one lemon's zest, flour, salt & lemon pepper.
- Add turkey & coat well.
- Bake turkey for 5 minutes with hot oil on one side.
- Add the rest of the ingredients with one lemon (in slices). Bake it until done and serve.

Nutrition: Kcal 231| Protein 14 g | Fiber 1.7 g | Carbs 12 g | Fat 6 g

18. Chicken Piccata

(Prep time: 10 minutes | Cook time: 20 minutes |Servings: 4)

Ingredients
- Granulated garlic, to taste
- 1 cup of all-purpose flour
- Salt & pepper, to taste
- 4 Tbsp. of olive oil
- 3 chicken breasts
- 2 Tbsp. of salted butter
- 2 garlic cloves, minced
- 1/4 cup of capers
- 1/3 cup of white wine
- 2 cups of chicken stock
- 2 lemons' juice
- 1 lemon, sliced

Instructions
- Slice the chicken into 6 cutlets season with granulated garlic, salt & pepper. Coat in flour.
- In a pan, add olive oil with butter (1 tbsp.), cook chicken for 4 minutes on 1 side. Take it out on a plate.

- In the same pan, brown the garlic in olive oil & butter. Add the slices of lemon, granulated garlic, salt, pepper, stock, lemon juice & wine.
- When it boils, add capers & chicken. Cook for 5 minutes. Serve.

Nutrition: Kcal 276 | Protein 17 g | Fiber 1 g | Carbs 14 g | Fat 15 g

19. Brazilian Fish Stew

(Prep time: 10 minutes | Cook time: 20 minutes |Servings: 4)

Ingredients

- 1 to 1 1/2 pounds of firm white fish
- One lime's juice & zest
- ½ tsp. of salt

Sauce

- 1 onion, diced
- 4 garlic cloves, chopped
- ½ tsp. of salt
- 2 to 3 tbsp. of olive oil
- 1 cup carrot, diced
- 1 red bell pepper, chopped
- ½ jalapeno, minced (optional)
- 1 cup of chicken stock
- 1 tbsp. of tomato paste
- ½ cup of chopped herbs
- 2 tsp. of paprika
- 1 tsp. of ground cumin
- 1 1/2 cups of chopped tomatoes
- 1 can of (14 oz.) coconut milk

Instructions

- Coat the fish in the lime juice (1 tbsp.), zest & salt.
- In a pan, sauté onion & salt for 2 to 3 minutes. Add jalapeno, carrot, garlic & bell pepper for 4 to 5 minutes.
- Add stock, spices & tomato paste. Simmer for 5 minutes.

- Add coconut milk salt. Stir & add fish; cook for 4 to 6 minutes.
- Adjust seasoning & serve.

Nutrition: Kcal 404 | Protein 44 g | Fiber 1.2 g | Carbs 12.6 g | Fat 19.7 g

20. Whole Roasted Trout

(Prep time: 10 minutes | Cook time: 20 minutes |Servings: 1-2)

Ingredients

- 1/2 lb. whole trout
- Salt & black pepper, to taste
- 1 lemon, sliced
- 6 sprigs of fresh thyme
- ½ shallot, thinly sliced
- 1/4 cup of walnuts halves
- 1 tbsp. of olive oil
- 4 tsp. butter, cubed

Instructions

- Let the oven preheat to 425°F.
- Coat the fish inside & outside with oil & season with salt & pepper.
- Place on an aluminum-lined baking tray with skin side down, add the rest of the ingredients on top, except for walnuts.
- Close the trout & bake for 12-16 minutes.
- Toast walnuts for 4-5 minutes & crush them.
- Fillet the cooked fish, top with crushed walnuts. Serve.

Nutrition: Kcal 178 | Protein 14.3 g | Fiber 2 g | Carbs 13 g | Fat 6 g

21. Garlic & Spinach Gnocchi

(Prep time: 10 minutes | Cook time: 40minutes |Servings: 4)

Ingredients

- 0.8 oz. of unsalted butter

- 3/4 cup of olive oil
- 1 bunch of spinach, chopped
- 1 cup of crumbled ricotta
- 1 garlic bulb
- ½ cup of grated parmesan
- 17 oz. of gnocchi
- 1 tbsp. of white wine vinegar

Instructions
- Let the oven preheat to 420°F.
- Coat the garlic bulb with oil & place on a foil piece & wrap in it.
- Roast for half an hour.
- Add the garlic cloves only to a processor, with oil, parmesan, spinach & salt. Pulse until smooth.
- Cook gnocchi as per package instructions, drain all but 1/3 cup of water.
- Add gnocchi to a pan with 2 tbsp. of oil & cook for 4 to 5 minutes.
- Add spinach sauce, gnocchi water & vinegar. Toss well.
- Serve.

Nutrition: Kcal 221 | Protein 9 g | Fiber 2 g | Carbs 15 g | Fat 2 g

22. Prawn & vegetable Pasta

(Prep time: 10 minutes | Cook time: 30minutes|Servings: 4)

Ingredients
- 3 tbsp. of olive oil
- 2 cups of baby spinach
- 2 minced garlic cloves
- 6 oz. of pasta
- ½ cup of fresh basil, sliced
- 1 tsp. of oregano
- 1.5 cups of cherry tomatoes
- 1 large zucchini, spiralized
- 18 medium prawns
- Salt & pepper, to taste

Instructions
- Cook pasta as per package instructions.
- Sauté oregano, olive oil & garlic for 1 minute. Add tomatoes & cook for 5 minutes.
- Add spinach cook until it wilts.
- In a different pan cook, the prawns with 1 tbsp. of oil for 1 to 2 minutes on one side. Turn the heat off.
- Add basil, zucchini noodles & pasta with spinach & tomatoes. Toss for 2 minutes.
- Adjust seasoning. Serve with prawns.

Nutrition: Kcal 246 | Protein 10 g | Fiber 3 g | Carbs 14 g | Fat 5 g

23. Turkey Quesadillas

(Prep time: 10 minutes | Cook time: 20minutes|Servings: 4)

Ingredients
- ½ onion, sliced
- Salt & pepper, to taste
- 1 lb. of turkey breasts, boneless & skinless strips
- 2 cups of shredded cheddar
- 2 bell peppers, sliced
- 1 tbsp. of vegetable oil
- 1 tbsp. of olive oil
- ½ tsp. of dried oregano
- 1 avocado, sliced
- ½ tsp. of ground cumin
- 4 flour tortillas
- 2 cups of Monterey jack, shredded

Instructions
- Sauté onion & peppers with salt & pepper for 5 minutes. Take it out on a plate.

- Season the turkey with salt, and pepper. Cook for 8 minutes & take it out on a plate.
- Warm the tortilla & top with cheese, onion, peppers & turkey with avocado slices & scallions.
- Fold & heat the tortillas for 3 minutes on each side.

Nutrition: Kcal 128 | Protein 7.9 g | Fiber 1 g | Carbs 13 g | Fat 7 g

24. Harvest Pizza

(Prep time: 10 minutes | Cook time: 15minutes|Servings: 2-3)

Ingredients

- 2 cloves garlic, sliced
- 1 ½ cups of fresh arugula
- 1 cup of red grapes, seedless & halved
- 1 Tbsp. of fresh rosemary
- 1 pizza crust (12")
- 4 Tbsp. olive oil
- One Pinch of crushed red pepper
- 1 Tbsp. of balsamic vinegar
- 1 cup of cooked chicken breast, shredded
- 1 cup of fennel bulb, sliced
- 1/3 cup of goat cheese, crumbled

Instructions

- Let the oven preheat to 425°F.
- Mix the oil, rosemary, red pepper & garlic. Microwave for 45 seconds.
- Season the chicken with 2 tbsp. Garlic oil. Place cheese, chicken, fennel & grapes on the crust.
- Bake for 10 minutes.
- Add vinegar to the rest of the garlic oil. Drizzle over pizza & serve.

Nutrition: Kcal 72 | Protein 0.1 g | Fiber 1.2 g | Carbs 18.7 g | Fat 0.2 g

25. Furikake Salmon

(Prep time: 10 minutes | Cook time: 15minutes|Servings: 2)

Ingredients

- 3 tbsp. of Mirin
- Salt, pepper, to taste
- 2 tbsp. of sesame oil
- 4 oz. of shiitake mushrooms, sliced without stems
- 2 tbsp. of olive oil
- 3 tbsp. of soy sauce
- 1 shallot, sliced
- 2 cups of shredded cabbage
- 8 to 10 oz. of salmon fillets

Instructions

- In a bowl, mix mirin, sesame oil & soy sauce.
- Sauté shallot & cabbage with salt & pepper until it wilts. Toss with a drizzle of soy sauce mixture.
- In a pan, add one tbsp. of oil. Add salt & pepper.
- Add mushrooms & salmon, cook on both sides. Add the soy sauce mixture.
- Serve the salmon with rice, cabbage & the rest of the ingredients.

Nutrition: Kcal 346| Protein 34 g | Fiber 3 g | Carbs 45 g | Fat 25 g

26. Maple-Mustard Chicken Leg

(Prep time: 10 minutes | Cook time: 45minutes|Servings: 4-6)

Ingredients

- 8 oz. of small carrots, cut in half
- 2 tbsp. of oil
- 12 oz. of baby potatoes, cut in half
- Salt & pepper, to taste
- 2 tbsp. of Dijon mustard
- 1 tsp. of fresh thyme leaves

- 4 whole chicken legs
- 2 tbsp. of whole-grain mustard
- 1 tbsp. of maple syrup

Instructions

- Let the oven preheat to 450°F.
- Toss carrots & potatoes with 1 tbsp. of oil, salt & pepper.
- Season the chicken with 1 tbsp. of oil, salt & pepper. Place on the baking dish skin side up with vegetables.
- Add the rest of the ingredients with a pinch of red pepper flakes.
- Brush the vegetables & chicken.
- Roast for 35 minutes. Brush with chicken juices & broil for 2-3 minutes. Serve.

Nutrition: Kcal 265 | Protein 21 g | Fiber 2 g | Carbs 13 g | Fat 8.1 g

27. Tandoori Chicken Skewers

(Prep time: 2 hours & 20 minutes | Cook time: 15minutes|Servings: 6)

Ingredients

- 1 cup of yogurt
- 2 tsp. of ground coriander
- 1 lemon's juice
- 18 chicken tenderloins, cut into smaller pieces
- 1 small onion, diced
- 6 cloves garlic, chopped
- 1 piece of (3") ginger, chopped
- 2 tsp. of ground cumin
- 1 tsp. of ground turmeric
- 1 tbsp. of garam masala
- 1 tsp. of kosher salt

Instructions

- In a bowl, add all ingredients except for chicken. Mix & add chicken, keep in the fridge for 2 hours.

- Thread the chicken onto soaked skewers and rest for half an hour at room temperature.
- Preheat the grill & oil spray the grates. Grill the skewers for 4-5 minutes on 1 side. Serve.

Nutrition: Kcal 156| Protein 23 g | Fiber 1 g | Carbs 8 g | Fat 8 g

28. Chicken, Mushroom & Avocado Fettuccine

(Prep time: 20 minutes | Cook time: 25minutes|Servings: 4)

Ingredients

- 17 oz. of chicken breast fillets
- 1 tbsp. of wholegrain mustard
- 14 oz. of mushrooms, sliced
- 2 garlic cloves, minced
- 1 1/2 tbsp. of olive oil
- Salt & pepper, to taste
- 1 cup of chicken stock
- 1 cup of cream
- 12 0z. of fettuccine
- 2 avocados, sliced
- 2 tbsp. of fresh dill sprigs

Instructions

- In a pan, heat 2 tsp. of oil.
- Season the chicken with salt & pepper.
- Cook in hot oil for 4 minutes on one side & take it out on a plate.
- Sauté the garlic & mushrooms for 5 to 6 minutes. Add mustard & cream.
- Let it come to a boil simmer for 12 to 15 minutes.
- Cook pasta as per package instructions. Add to the pan.
- Toss & serve with sliced chicken & avocado.

Nutrition: Kcal 309| Protein 23 g | Fiber 1 g | Carbs 20 g | Fat 16 g

29. Chicken Noodle Soup

(Prep time: 20 minutes | Cook time: 6 hours | Servings: 6)

Ingredients

- 3 celery stalks, sliced
- 1 tbsp. of thyme
- 3 carrots, sliced
- 1 onion, diced
- 1 lb. chicken breast, boneless & skinless
- 2 minced garlic cloves
- 8 cups of chicken stock
- 1 tbsp. of rosemary
- 1 tsp. of salt
- 8 oz. of egg noodles

Instructions

- Add all ingredients to a slow cooker, except
- Cook for 6 to 8 hours on low or 3 to 4 hours on high.
- In the last 14 minutes, take the chicken out & shred it.
- Add to the cooker with noodles. Cook for 14-15 minutes. Serve.

Nutrition: Kcal 276| Protein 24 g | Fiber 1 g | Carbs 15 g | Fat 6.2 g

Chapter 6: HIGH FIBER RECIPES

6.1 BREAKFAST

1. Cherry-Mocha Smoothie

(Prep time: 20 minutes | Cook time: 0minutes|Servings: 6)

Ingredients

- 1 cup of almond Choco milk, unsweetened
- 1 tsp. of instant coffee
- 5.3 to 6-oz. of Greek yogurt
- 1 tsp. of vanilla
- ½ banana
- 1 cup of frozen dark cherries, unsweetened & pitted
- 2 tbsp. of cocoa powder, unsweetened
- 2 tbsp. of almond butter
- 2 cups of ice cubes

Instructions

- Add all ingredients to a blender. Pulse until smooth.
- Serve by pouring in a chilled glass.

Nutrition: Kcal 272 | Protein 13 g | Fiber 8 g | Carbs 34 g | Fat 12 g

2. Pumpkin Overnight Oats

(Prep time: Overnight & 10 minutes | Cook time: 0minutes|Servings: 2)

Ingredients

- 1/4 cup of plain yogurt
- 2/3 cup of almond milk, unsweetened
- 1/4 cup of pumpkin puree
- 1 packet of instant oats
- 1 tsp. of maple syrup
- Half tsp. of pumpkin pie spice

Instructions

- In a mason jar, add all ingredients. Shake well & keep in the fridge overnight.
- Serve.

Nutrition: Kcal 190| Protein 5 g | Fiber 6 g | Carbs 32 g | Fat 4 g

3. Breakfast Bars

(Prep time: 20 minutes | Cook time: 30minutes|Servings: 12)

Ingredients

- ¼ cup of wheat germ
- ¼ cup of ground flax seed
- ¼ cup + ¼ cup of peanut butter
- 3 bananas
- 2 tbsp. of hemp protein powder (vanilla-flavored)
- 1 tsp. of ground cinnamon
- 1 ½ cups of quick-cooking oats
- 1 tsp. of vanilla extract
- Half tsp. of salt
- 2 tbsp. of honey

Instructions

- Let the oven preheat to 375°F.
- Line an 8 by 8 baking dish with aluminum
- In a bowl, mix salt, flax seed, cinnamon, wheat germ, protein powder & oats.
- In a bowl, mash bananas with peanut butter (1/4 cup), honey & vanilla extract.
- Add to the dry ingredients & mix.
- Bake for 20 minutes, add peanut butter on top & spread.

- Bake for 10 minutes.
- Slice & serve.

Nutrition: Kcal 87| Protein 6 g | Fiber 6 g | Carbs 11 g | Fat 5 g

4. Chocolate Smoothie

(Prep time: 20 minutes | Cook time: 0minutes|Servings: 12)

Ingredients
- ¼ cup of Cacao Bliss
- 2 cups of milk
- ¼ cup of almond butter
- Ice
- 2 bananas, sliced & frozen
- 2 tbsp. of hemp hearts

Instructions
- Add all ingredients to a blender. Pulse until smooth.
- Serve by pouring in a chilled glass.

Nutrition: Kcal 515| Protein 22 g | Fiber 11 g | Carbs 48 g | Fat 31 g

5. Sweet Potato Waffles

(Prep time: 20 minutes | Cook time: 30minutes|Servings: 12)

Ingredients
- ½ cup of Rolled Oats
- 1/4 Cup of maple syrup
- ½ cup of Sweet Potato pureed
- 2 Eggs
- 1 Tsp. of Cinnamon
- 1 Cup of Whole Wheat Flour
- 1/2 cup Almond Milk, Unsweetened
- 2 Tsp. of Baking Powder
- 1/4 Tsp. of Salt

Instructions
- In a bowl, add all the dry ingredients.
- Mix & add the wet ingredients. Mix & pour on the heated waffle iron.
- Cook & serve.

Nutrition: Kcal 212 | Protein 3 g | Fiber 5 g | Carbs 12 g | Fat 6 g

6. Chocolate Buckwheat Waffles

(Prep time: 20 minutes | Cook time: 30minutes|Servings: 6)

Ingredients
- 9 tbsp. of sugar
- ¾ tsp. of baking soda
- 1/2cup of yogurt
- ¾ tsp. of vanilla extract
- 4 ½ cups of quartered strawberries
- 1 tbsp. of oil
- 4 ½ oz. of buckwheat flour
- ⅓ cup of unsweetened cocoa
- ⅛ tsp. of salt
- 1 ¼ cups of buttermilk
- 3 egg whites
- ¼ cup of water
- 2 egg yolks
- 2 tbsp. of sliced almonds, toasted

Instructions
- Toss the strawberries with 2 tbsp. of sugar. Let it rest for half an hour.
- Mix yogurt with ¼ tsp. of vanilla & sugar (1 tbsp.) mix & keep in the fridge.
- In a bowl, whisk salt, flour, baking soda & cocoa.
- Add vanilla (half tsp.), yolks, buttermilk, whisk & add to the flour.
- Heat the waffle iron.
- Whisk the egg white until foamy, add sugar (6 tbsp.) gradually whisk until peaks form.
- Fold the egg whites into the mixture. Pour on the waffle iron & cook for 4 minutes.
- Serve.

Nutrition: Kcal 267 | Protein 11 g | Fiber 7 g | Carbs 27 g | Fat 1.3 g

7. Banana-Nut Oatmeal Cups

(Prep time: 25 minutes | Cook time: 30minutes|Servings: 12)

Ingredients

- 1 ½ cups of milk
- 1 tsp. of baking powder
- 1 tsp. of vanilla extract
- 2 bananas, mashed
- 3 cups of rolled oats
- ⅓ cup of packed brown sugar
- 2 eggs, whisked
- ½ cup of chopped pecans, toasted
- 1 tsp. of ground cinnamon
- Half tsp. of salt

Instructions

- Let the oven preheat to 375°F
- Add all ingredients to a bowl, mix & pour in the oil sprayed muffin tin.
- Bake for 25 minutes and then serve.

Nutrition: Kcal 176 | Protein 5.2 g | Fiber 4 g | Carbs 26.4 g | Fat 6.2 g

8. Breakfast Salad

(Prep time: 25 minutes | Cook time: 5minutes|Servings: 1)

Ingredients

- 1 tbsp. + 1 tsp. olive oil
- 8 blue corn tortilla chips, chopped up
- ¼ avocado, sliced
- 2 tbsp. of chopped cilantro
- 3 tbsp. of salsa verde
- 2 cups of salad greens
- ½ cup of canned kidney beans, rinsed
- 1 egg

Instructions

- Mix cilantro, salsa & one tbsp. of oil. Add the salad greens & toss.
- Add the avocado, beans & chips on top.
- Fry eggs in one tsp. of oil for 2 minutes.
- Serve the salad with an egg on top.

Nutrition: Kcal 527| Protein 16 g | Fiber 13 g | Carbs 37 g | Fat 30 g

9. Muesli with Raspberries

(Prep time: 5 minutes | Cook time: 0minutes|Servings: 1)

Ingredients

- ⅓ cup of muesli
- ¾ cup of milk
- 1 cup of raspberries

Instructions

- Serve with milk, with muesli & raspberries.

Nutrition: Kcal 288| Protein 13 g | Fiber 13 g | Carbs 51 g | Fat 6.6 g

10. Spinach & Egg Scramble

(Prep time: 25 minutes | Cook time: 6-8minutes|Servings: 1)

Ingredients

- 1 tsp. of canola oil
- 1 slice of toasted whole-grain bread
- ½ cup of fresh raspberries
- 1 ½ cups of baby spinach
- 2 eggs, whisked
- Salt & pepper, to taste

Instructions

- Sauté spinach in hot oil for 1-2 minutes. Take it out on a plate.
- Add eggs & cook for 1-2 minutes until set; add the spinach.
- Adjust seasoning. Serve on toast, topped with raspberries.

Nutrition: Kcal 296 | Protein 17.8 g | Fiber 8 g | Carbs 20 g | Fat 15 g

11. Apple-Cinnamon Oats

(Prep time: 10 minutes | Cook time: 0minutes|Servings: 1)

Ingredients

- 1/4 cup of yogurt
- Half tsp. of pumpkin pie spice
- 1/4 cup of pumpkin puree
- 2/3 cup of almond milk, unsweetened
- 1 packet of instant oats
- 1 tsp. of maple syrup

Instructions

- In a mason jar, add all ingredients. Shake well & keep in the fridge overnight.
- Serve.

Nutrition: Kcal 190| Protein 5 g | Fiber 6 g | Carbs 32 g | Fat 4 g

12. PB&J Smoothie

(Prep time: 10 minutes | Cook time: 0minutes|Servings: 1)

Ingredients

- 1 cup of frozen strawberries
- 1 tsp. of honey
- ¼ cup of rolled oats
- 1 banana, sliced
- 2 tbsp. of almond butter
- 1 tbsp. of chia seeds
- ½ cup of almond milk, unsweetened

Instructions

- In a mason jar, add all ingredients. Shake well & keep in the fridge overnight.
- Serve.

Nutrition: Kcal 89| Protein 3.4 g | Fiber 6 g | Carbs 13 g | Fat 1.2 g

13. Strawberry Banana Overnight Oats

(Prep time: 10 minutes | Cook time: 0minutes|Servings: 1)

Ingredients

- 1/4 Cup of Yogurt
- ½ cup of Vanilla Almond Milk, unsweetened
- Half cup of rolled Oats
- 1 Scoop of Protein Powder (Vanilla)
- Half ripe Banana, Mashed
- 1 Tbsp. of Ground Flaxseed
- 1/3 Cup of Strawberries, Freeze Dried

Instructions

- In a mason jar, add all ingredients. Shake well & keep in the fridge overnight.
- Serve.

Nutrition: Kcal 97| Protein 4.1 g | Fiber 5.9 g | Carbs 12 g | Fat 2.1 g

14. Sweet Corn Oatmeal

(Prep time: 10 minutes | Cook time: 10minutes|Servings: 4)

Ingredients

- 2 cups of corn kernels
- 1 tbsp. of maple syrup
- 1 cup of milk
- ⅛ tsp. of ground nutmeg
- 2 cups of rolled oats
- 1 tbsp. of unsalted butter
- 1 tsp. of kosher salt
- ¼ tsp. of vanilla extract
- 3 cups of water
- ¼ cup of yogurt
- 1 cup of sliced peaches

Instructions

- In a pan, heat butter, cook corn syrup for 3 minutes.
- Add salt & oats. Cook for 2 minutes.
- Add milk, water & nutmeg, cook for 5 minutes.
- Add vanilla & yogurt mix.

- Divide the oats into 4 bowls, top with yogurt & serve.

Nutrition: Kcal 314| Protein 11 g | Fiber 6 g | Carbs 51 g | Fat 1.6 g

15. Peanut Butter & Chia Jam

(Prep time: 10 minutes | Cook time: 2minutes|Servings: 1)

Ingredients

- 1 toasted English muffin
- 2 tsp. of chia seeds
- Half cup of mixed frozen berries
- 2 tsp. of peanut butter

Instructions

- Add berries to a bowl & microwave for 30 seconds. Stir & add chia seeds.
- Serve the muffin, topped with peanut butter & berry jam.

Nutrition: Kcal 262 | Protein 9.8 g | Fiber 9.4 g | Carbs 40 g | Fat 9 g

16. Coconut-Green Apple Muesli

(Prep time: 10 minutes | Cook time: 0minutes|Servings: 4)

Ingredients

- ½ cup of coconut milk, unsweetened
- 1/8 tsp. of kosher salt
- 1/4 cup of orange juice
- 1 1/2 cups of coconut yogurt, unsweetened
- 2 tbsp. of maple syrup
- 1 apple, cored & shredded
- 1/4 tsp. of ground cinnamon
- 1 cup of rolled oats
- ½ cup of unsweetened coconut, shredded

Instructions

- Mix all liquid ingredients add the rest of the ingredients.
- Serve chilled.

Nutrition: Kcal 315 | Protein 6 g | Fiber 10 g | Carbs 41 g | Fat 16 g

17. Freezer Breakfast Burritos

(Prep time: 10 minutes | Cook time: 12minutes|Servings: 6)

Ingredients

- 1 pack of 14 oz. extra-firm tofu, crumbled
- 1 cup of corn
- 6 whole-wheat (8") tortillas
- 1 tsp. of ground cumin
- 2 tbsp. of oil
- ¼ cup of fresh cilantro
- ¼ tsp. of salt
- 1 can of 15 oz. black beans, rinsed
- 4 scallions, sliced
- ½ cup of salsa

Instructions

- Sauté the tofu with salt in hot oil (1 tbsp.) for 10-12 minutes. Take it out in a bowl.
- Add more oil with scallions, beans & corn cook for 3 minutes.
- Add tofu back to the pan with salsa. Cook for 2 minutes.
- Serve in warm tortillas after rolling the tortilla. Or freeze for up to three months.

Nutrition: Kcal 329 | Protein 15 g | Fiber 7.7 g | Carbs 44 g | Fat 10 g

18. Quinoa Breakfast Bars

(Prep time: 10 minutes | Cook time: 20minutes|Servings: 6)

Ingredients

- 1.5 cups of cooked quinoa
- 1 tsp. of baking soda
- 2 cups of oats
- 1 cup of whole wheat flour
- ½ cup of nuts, chopped

- ½ cup of honey
- 1 tsp. of cinnamon
- 2/3 cup of peanut butter
- 1/3 cup of raisins
- 2 eggs
- 2/3 cup of applesauce
- 2 Tbsp. of chia seeds
- 1 tsp. of vanilla
- ½ tsp. of salt

Instructions

- In a bowl, mix honey, quinoa, eggs, applesauce, peanut butter & vanilla.
- Add the rest of the ingredients & mix.
- Oil spray a 9 by 13" baking sheet. Add the mixture & bake for 20 minutes at 375°F.
- Cool, slice & serve.

Nutrition: Kcal 215| Protein 9 g | Fiber 12 g | Carbs 16 g | Fat 7 g

19. Chocolate Chip Zucchini Bread

(Prep time: 10 minutes | Cook time: 30minutes|Servings: 6)

Ingredients

- 3/4 Cup of Coconut Sugar
- ½ cup of melted Coconut Oil
- 3 eggs
- ½ tsp. of Baking Soda
- 1 Tsp. of Vanilla Extract
- ½ tsp. of Baking Powder
- 1 Cup of Chocolate Chips
- 2 Cups of Whole Wheat Pastry Flour
- 1 Tsp. of Salt
- 2 Cups of Shredded Zucchini, squeezed

Instructions

- Let the oven preheat to 350°F.
- Oil spray small loaf pans.
- Whisk eggs with vanilla, sugar & oil until smooth.

- Add the dry ingredients & mix.
- Add chocolate chips & zucchini, add to the small loaf pans.
- Bake the small loaf pans for 30 to 35 minutes.
- Serve.

Nutrition: Kcal 165 | Protein 8.1 g | Fiber 8.7 g | Carbs 16.9 g | Fat 8 g

20. Apple-Oat Energy Balls

(Prep time: 10 minutes | Cook time: 0minutes|Servings: 6)

Ingredients

- 1 tsp. of kosher salt
- 1 cup of grated apple
- 2 ½ cups of rolled oats
- ½ cup of shredded coconut, unsweetened
- ¼ cup of honey
- ½ cup of almond butter
- 1 tsp. of ground cinnamon

Instructions

- In a food processor, add all ingredients. Pulse until smooth.
- Make it into 12 balls.
- Serve chilled.

Nutrition: Kcal 72 | Protein 5 g | Fiber 10 g | Carbs 9 g | Fat 6 g

21. Blueberry Muffins

(Prep time: 10 minutes | Cook time: 30minutes|Servings: 12)

Ingredients

- ¼ cup of coconut flour
- 1 cup of blueberries
- 1 tbsp. of baking powder
- 1 ½ tsp. of vanilla extract
- 1 ¾ cups of almond flour
- ¼ tsp. of baking soda
- ¼ tsp. of salt

- ⅓ cup + 2 tbsp. of light brown sugar
- 3 eggs
- Half cups of milk
- ¼ cup of avocado oil

Instructions

- Let the oven preheat to 350°F.
- Oil spray a muffin tin.
- Add all dry ingredients to a bowl & mix.
- Add all dry ingredients to a bowl & mix.
- Fold in blueberries mix the wet to dry ingredients.
- Add in muffin cups.
- Bake for 20-15 minutes.

Nutrition: Kcal 204 | Protein 5.8 g | Fiber 2.9 g | Carbs 15 g | Fat 14 g

22. Strawberry, Blueberry & Banana Smoothie

(Prep time: 10 minutes | Cook time: 0minutes|Servings: 1)

Ingredients

- Half cup of frozen blueberries
- 1 tbsp. of cashew butter
- 1 frozen ripe banana
- 1 tbsp. of hulled hemp seeds
- Half cup of frozen strawberries
- ¾ cup of chilled cashew milk, unsweetened

Instructions

- Add all ingredients to a blender. Pulse until smooth.
- Serve by pouring in a chilled glass.

Nutrition: Kcal 335 | Protein 6 g | Fiber 8 g | Carbs 45 g | Fat 16 g

23. Banana Buckwheat Pancakes

(Prep time: 10 minutes | Cook time: 10minutes|Servings: 2-3)

Ingredients

- 1 banana, mashed
- 1 tsp. of baking soda
- ½ cup of almond milk, unsweetened
- 2 tsp. of cinnamon
- 1 ½ cups of buckwheat flour
- 2 eggs
- 1 tsp. of vanilla extract

Instructions

- Add all ingredients to a bowl & mix well.
- Add to a heated pan in butter, cook on both sides until golden brown & serve.

Nutrition: Kcal 189 | Protein 09 g | Fiber 11 g | Carbs 19 g | Fat 3.4 g

24. Blue Corn Waffles Rancheros

(Prep time: 10 minutes | Cook time: 50minutes|Servings: 4)

Ingredients

Chipotle Aioli

- 1 egg yolk
- ¼ cup of avocado oil
- ¼ cup of chipotle peppers in adobo
- ⅛ tsp. of salt
- 1 tsp. of lemon juice
- 1 clove garlic, diced

Tomatillo Salsa

- 1 onion, thickly sliced
- ⅛ tsp. of salt
- ½ jalapeño pepper (optional)
- 8 oz. of tomatillos
- 1 clove garlic
- 1 tbsp. of chopped fresh cilantro

Waffles & Topping

- ½ cup of masa harina
- 2 tsp. of baking powder
- 1 ¼ cups of blue cornmeal
- ¼ tsp. of salt
- 5 eggs

- 1 cup of milk
- 3 tbsp. butter, melted
- 1 can (15 oz.) black beans, rinsed
- 1 ½ tsp. of maple syrup
- 1 tbsp. of avocado oil

Instructions
- In a food processor, add all ingredients of aioli except for oil.
- While running the machine, add the oil slowly & set it aside.
- Place jalapenos, onion, peeled garlic & tomatillos on a baking sheet & broil for 10 minutes, turning as needed.
- Cool for a few minutes, add to a food processor with the rest of the ingredients. Pulse until chopped.
- Let the oven preheat to 200°F.
- For waffles, add dry & wet ingredients (except for beans) to different bowls & whisk.
- Add the wet to dry ingredients.
- Cook waffles on a waffle iron for 2-4 minutes.
- Serve the waffles with aioli, beans & salsa.

Nutrition: Kcal 706 | Protein 23 g | Fiber 12 g | Carbs 69 g | Fat 38 g

25. Apple Flax Breakfast Squares

(Prep time: 10 minutes | Servings: 12)

Ingredients
- 2 tsp. of baking powder
- 2 tsp. of cinnamon
- 3 cups of ground flaxseed
- ½ cup of apple sauce, unsweetened
- ½ tsp. of nutmeg
- ½ tsp. of salt
- ½ cup of walnuts, chopped
- ½ cup of maple syrup
- 1 apple, chopped

- 4 eggs
- 2 tsp. of vanilla extract
- ¼ cup plus 1 tsp. of melted coconut oil

Instructions
- Let the oven preheat to 350°F. Oil spray a 9 by 13" pan.
- Mix the wet & dry ingredients in 2 different bowls.
- Mix the wet in dry ingredients.
- Spread on the oil sprayed pan. Bake for half an hour.
- Slice & serve.

Nutrition: Kcal 286 | Protein 9 g | Fiber 9 g | Carbs 13g | Fat 20 g

26. Strawberry Cheesecake Oats

(Prep time: 10 minutes | Servings: 3)

Ingredients
- 1/3 Cup of Fresh Strawberries, chopped
- 10 oz. of Vanilla Protein Shake
- 1 ½ Cups of Oats
- 5 oz. of Strawberry Yogurt
- 2 Tbsp. of Chia Seeds

Instructions
- Add all ingredients to a mason jar. Shake well & keep in the fridge overnight.
- Serve.

Nutrition: Kcal 103 | Protein 4 g | Fiber 8 g | Carbs 12 g | Fat 2 g

27. Banana-Chocolate French Toast

(Prep time: 15 minutes | Cook time: 6minutes|Servings: 3)

Ingredients
- 2 eggs, whisked
- ⅛ tsp. of salt
- ¾ tsp. of vanilla extract
- ¼ cup of milk

- ½ tsp. of sugar
- 1 cup of sliced thin banana
- 6 slices of whole-grain bread
- 1 ½ tsp. of powdered sugar
- 4 ½ tbsp. of Nutella spread
- 2 tsp. of canola oil

Instructions
- Add 5 first ingredients in a bowl & mix.
- Spread Nutella on 3 bread slices, place banana slices on top.
- Place the 3 slices on top.
- Heat oil in a skillet. Add the sandwiches to the milk mixture & flip to coat well.
- Add to the pan cook for 2 minutes on one side.
- Slice & serve.

Nutrition: Kcal 390 | Protein 5 g | Fiber 6 g | Carbs 53 g | Fat 13.8 g

28. Breakfast Sandwich

(Prep time: 10 minutes | Cook time: 0minutes|Servings: 1)

Ingredients
- 1 toasted bagel thin
- 1 slice of Monterey Jack cheese
- 2 tbsp. of sliced thinly red onion
- ¼ avocado, sliced
- 1 tbsp. of garlic mayonnaise
- 2 tbsp. of alfalfa sprouts
- 1 fried egg

Instructions
- In between the bagel, add the rest of the ingredients.
- Top with the other half & serve.

Nutrition: Kcal 492| Protein 19 g | Fiber 9 g | Carbs 30 g | Fat 36 g

29. Mocha Protein Overnight Oats

(Prep time: 10 minutes | Servings: 2)

Ingredients
- 1 ¼ Cup of Unsweetened Vanilla Almond Milk
- 1 Tsp. of Vanilla Extract
- 1 ½ Tbsp. of Chia Seeds
- 1 Cup of rolled Oats
- 1 Scoop of Coffee Protein Powder
- 1 Tbsp. of Cocoa Powder
- 1 Tsp. of Cinnamon
- 2 Tsp. of maple syrup

Instructions
- In a mason jar, add all ingredients. Shake well & keep in the fridge overnight.
- Serve.

Nutrition: Kcal 190| Protein 5 g | Fiber 6 g | Carbs 32 g | Fat 4 g

30. Avocado Matcha Banana Bread

(Prep time: 10 minutes /Servings: 1 loaf)

Ingredients
- 1 ½ cups of all-purpose flour
- 1 egg
- 1 ½ tbsp. of matcha powder
- 1 teaspoon vanilla extract
- 1 tsp. of baking soda
- ½ tsp. of kosher salt
- 2 tsp. of black sesame seeds
- ¾ cup of granulated sugar
- 1 avocado
- 2 ripe bananas
- ¼ cup of vegetable oil

Instructions
- Let the oven preheat to 350°F. Oil spray a 9 by 5" loaf pan.
- Add all dry ingredients to a bowl & mix.
- Add egg, avocado & vanilla to a food processor & pulse until smooth.
- Mash the bananas. Mix with oil & avocado mixture.

- Add the wet to dry ingredients.
- Pour in a pan sprinkle with black seeds.

- Bake for 50 to 55 minutes.

Nutrition: Kcal 276 | Protein 6 g | Fiber 8 g | Carbs 14 g | Fat 6 g

6.2 LUNCH

1. Super-Greens Frittata

(Prep time: 10 minutes | Cook time: 20minutes|Servings: 4)

Ingredients

- Half cup of fresh parsley
- 2.82 oz. of baby spinach
- 3 scallions, chopped
- 1 cup of fresh basil
- 1 tbsp. of lemon zest
- 2 zucchinis, roughly chopped
- 2 tbsp. of olive oil
- 7 oz. of broccoli, broken into florets
- 8 eggs
- Half cup of yogurt
- 8.8 oz. of mixed mushrooms, sliced
- 2 garlic cloves, sliced

Instructions

- In a food processor, add scallions, basil, spinach, zucchini & parsley. Pulse until chopped.
- In a pan, add half of the oil & add the parsley mixture; cook for 5 minutes.
- Whisk yogurt with eggs, salt & pepper. Add to the pan.
- Cook for 8-10 minutes on low flame, until almost set.
- In a pan, sauté mushrooms & broccoli in the rest of the oil.
- Cook for 6 minutes.
- Add the lemon zest & garlic, cook for 1 minute. Turn the heat off.

- Broil the frittata for 2 minutes, serve with garlic mixture on top.

Nutrition: Kcal 412 | Protein 7 g | Fiber 9 g | Carbs 6 g | Fat 26 g

2. Satisfying Salad

(Prep time: 15 minutes | Cook time: 0minutes|Servings: 3)

Ingredients

- 1 onion
- 1 garlic clove
- 10 walnuts, chopped
- 1 cup of sliced cabbage
- Half lemon's juice
- 1 cup of sliced lettuce
- 10 olives
- 1 red pepper
- 1 cup of canned white beans
- 1 tsp. of balsamic vinegar
- Half cup of canned corn
- 1 carrot
- 1 tbsp. of olive oil

Instructions

Chop the vegetables to your liking.

Add all the ingredients to a bowl, mix well & serve.

Adjust seasoning & serve.

Nutrition: Kcal 383 | Protein 13 g | Fiber 10 g | Carbs 38 g | Fat 23 g

3. Roasted Chicken & Winter Squash Salad

(Prep time: 15 minutes | Cook time: 25minutes|Servings: 4)

Ingredients

- 3 tbsp. of olive oil
- 2 tbsp. of lemon juice
- 2 tbsp. of whole-grain mustard
- 3 minced cloves of garlic
- 2 ½ pounds of delicata squash
- 4 tsp. of grated Parmesan cheese
- 4 tsp. of roasted pumpkin seeds
- 1 tbsp. of fresh rosemary, chopped
- 1 tsp. of lemon zest
- 1 tbsp. of maple syrup
- 1 tsp. of black pepper
- Half tsp. of salt
- 8 cups of mixed salad greens
- 1 pound of chicken breast, boneless & skinless
- 1 ½ tsp. of fresh thyme leaves

Instructions

- Let the oven preheat to 425 F.
- Slice the squash in half & take the seeds out. Slice into one" slice.
- In a bowl, mix salt (1/4 tsp.), oil (1 tbsp.), rosemary, zest, black pepper (half tsp.), mustard (1 1/2 tbsp.), lemon juice (half tbsp.) & garlic.
- Add squash & chicken, coat well.
- Spread on a baking sheet. Bake for 20-23 minutes without stirring.
- Add the rest of the ingredients to a bowl toss to coat.
- Serve the greens with sliced chicken & squash.

Nutrition: Kcal 415 | Protein 31 g | Fiber 7.2 g | Carbs 38 g | Fat 16 g

4. Cauliflower & Oat Soup with Turmeric

(Prep time: 15 minutes | Cook time: 60minutes|Servings: 4)

Ingredients

- 4 cups of cauliflower florets
- 1 onion, cut into quarters
- 1 tbsp. of olive oil
- 1 cup of Quick Oats
- 2 celery stalks, chopped large
- 1 1/2 tsp. of ground turmeric
- 4 cups of vegetable broth
- 1 1/2 tsp. of thyme leaves, crushed
- Half tsp. of salt
- Black pepper, to taste
- 1 tsp. of grated ginger

Instructions

- Let the oven preheat to 450 F.
- Oil spray a sheet of aluminum sheet.
- Pulse the half cup of oats in the food processor.
- In a bowl, add onion, cauliflower & celery.
- Whisk the oil, turmeric, salt & thyme. Pour on the vegetables & toss.
- Spread the vegetables on the baking sheets sprinkle black pepper.
- Roast for 15 minutes, stir & roast for 10-16 minutes more.
- Add to a food processor, with a half cup of broth & ginger.
- Pulse until smooth, add to a pan.
- Add the broth & pulsed oats. Simmer for 15 minutes.
- Add whole oats cook for 3 to 5 minutes.
- Add more water if necessary, serve.

Nutrition: Kcal 181 | Protein 6.9 g | Fiber 7 g | Carbs 28 g | Fat 5 g

5. Red Lentil Soup

(Prep time: 15 minutes | Cook time: 40minutes|Servings: 4)

Ingredients

- 1 onion, chopped
- 1 cup of dry red lentils
- 1 tbsp. of minced ginger
- 1 chopped clove garlic
- 1 tbsp. of peanut oil
- 1 pinch of fenugreek seeds
- Half can of (14 oz.) coconut milk
- 1 cup of peeled & cubed butternut squash
- ⅓ cup of fresh cilantro, chopped
- 1 pinch of each nutmeg & cayenne pepper
- 2 cups of water
- 1 tsp. of curry powder
- Salt & pepper, to taste
- 2 tbsp. of tomato paste

Instructions

- Sauté the onion, garlic, fenugreek & ginger in hot oil until tender.
- Add cilantro, lentils & squash in a pot.
- Add tomato paste, water & coconut milk with seasonings.
- Let it come to a boil, turn the heat low and simmer for half an hour.

Nutrition: Kcal 303 | Protein 13 g | Fiber 1.2 g | Carbs 34 g | Fat 14 g

6. Mediterranean Chicken Noodle Soup

(Prep time: 15 minutes | Cook time: 4 hours |Servings: 6)

Ingredients

- 4 cups of chicken broth
- 1 ½ cups of diced yellow onion
- 1 pound of chicken breast, boneless & skinless

- Half tsp. of black pepper
- 1 can of (14 oz.) fire-roasted diced tomatoes
- 6 oz. of whole-wheat rotini pasta
- 1 cup of diced bell pepper
- 4 minced cloves garlic
- 1 tbsp. of Italian seasoning
- Half cup of grated Parmesan cheese
- ¼ tsp. of each salt & red pepper flakes
- 1 bay leaf
- 2 tbsp. of fresh basil, chopped
- 2 tbsp. of parsley

Instructions

- In a slow cooker, add all ingredients except for herbs & pasta.
- Cook for 3 hours on high.
- Take the chicken out add pasta & herbs. Cook for half an hour more.
- Shred the chicken add it back to the pot, heat it through & serve.

Nutrition: Kcal 256 | Protein 23 g | Fiber 6 g | Carbs 29 g | Fat 4.6 g

7. Pasta with Green Peas

(Prep time: 15 minutes | Cook time: 30minutes|Servings: 4)

Ingredients

- 2 Garlic Cloves
- Half tsp. of Nutmeg
- 12 oz. of Whole Wheat Penne Pasta
- 11 oz. of Peas
- 12 oz. of Broccoli Florets
- 2 tbsp. of Olive Oil
- 4 tbsp. of Fresh Parsley

Instructions

- Sauté the garlic & nutmeg in hot oil for 30 seconds.
- Add the parsley, peas & florets with a splash of water, cook for 10 minutes.
- Add salt & pepper.

- Cook pasta as per package instructions. Drain & add to the sauce with some of the pasta water.
- Toss well & serve.

Nutrition: Kcal 276 | Protein 6 g | Fiber 6.2 g | Carbs 19 g | Fat 5 g

8. High Fiber Pasta

(Prep time: 15 minutes | Cook time: 45minutes|Servings: 6)

Ingredients

- 17 oz. of pumpkin, peeled & cubes
- 1 tsp. of olive oil
- ¼ cup of fresh basil, sliced
- 1 garlic clove, minced
- 17 oz. of Whole Meal Spaghetti
- 4 red capsicums, cut into fours without seeds
- 4.4 oz. of olives, halved
- 7 oz. of feta, crumbled
- Salt & black pepper

Instructions

- Let the oven preheat to 390 F.
- Oil spray 2 baking trays.
- In a bowl, toss pumpkin & garlic with oil, salt & pepper. Roast for half an hour on one tray.
- On the other tray, add capsicum & bake for half an hour.
- Cook pasta as per package instructions.
- Slice the capsicum & mix with pasta with the rest of the ingredients.
- Add salt & pepper. Serve.

Nutrition: Kcal 323 | Protein 5 g | Fiber 8 g | Carbs 14 g | Fat 6 g

9. Salmon-Stuffed Avocados

(Prep time: 15 minutes | Cook time: 0minutes|Servings: 4)

Ingredients

- Half cup of diced celery
- 2 cans of (5 oz. each) salmon, without skin & bones, drained
- ⅛ tsp. of each salt & pepper
- 2 tbsp. of fresh parsley, chopped
- 1 tbsp. of lime juice
- Half cup of Greek yogurt
- 2 tsp. of mayonnaise
- 1 tsp. of Dijon mustard
- 2 avocados

Instructions

- Cut the avocados in half, take the flesh out & leave the bowls.
- Add to a bowl (only half the flesh) with the rest of the ingredients, mix & stuff in the avocado shells.
- Serve.

Nutrition: Kcal 293| Protein 22 g | Fiber 7 g | Carbs 10 g | Fat 18 g

10. Honey Mustard Salmon

(Prep time: 15 minutes | Cook time: 10minutes|Servings: 4)

Ingredients

- Salt & Pepper to taste
- 2 tbsp. of Honey
- 4 Salmon Filets
- 2 tbsp. of Dijon Mustard
- Small lemon's juice

Instructions

- In a bowl, add all ingredients except for fish. Mix.
- Add fish & coat well.
- Broil the fish for 5 minutes on each side, serve with salad greens.

Nutrition: Kcal 176 | Protein 8 g | Fiber 4.2 g | Carbs 5 g | Fat 4 g

11. Lamb Dhal Makhani

(Prep time: 15 minutes | Cook time: 30minutes|Servings: 4)

Ingredients

- 1 brown onion, chopped
- 10 oz. of lamb mince
- 2 tsp. of ground cumin
- 14 oz. of canned red kidney beans, rinsed
- 1 tbsp. of vegetable oil
- 1-inch piece of fresh ginger, grated
- 14 oz. of canned lentils, rinsed
- 2 garlic cloves, minced
- 1 cinnamon stick
- 2 tbsp. of tomato paste
- 14 oz. of can tomato puree

Instructions

- Sauté the onion & mince in hot oil for 6-8 minutes.
- Add cumin, garlic, ginger & cinnamon. Cook for 1 minute.
- Add tomato paste cook for 2 minutes. Add the rest of the ingredients to boil.
- Simmer for 10 minutes. Discard the cinnamon & serve.

Nutrition: Kcal 245 | Protein 9 g | Fiber 7 g | Carbs 13 g | Fat 4 g

12. Classic Sesame Noodles

(Prep time: 15 minutes | Cook time: 15minutes|Servings: 4)

Ingredients

- 3 tbsp. of dark sesame oil
- 1 tsp. of brown sugar
- 2 scallions, sliced
- 1 tbsp. of minced garlic
- 1 cup of julienned carrots
- 8 oz. of whole-wheat spaghetti
- 2 tsp. of minced ginger
- 2 tbsp. of soy sauce
- 3 tbsp. of toasted sesame seeds

- 2 tbsp. of ketchup
- 8 oz. of cooked & shredded chicken breast, boneless & skinless
- 1 cup of snap peas, sliced

Instructions

- Cook noodles as per package instructions.
- Drain & add to a bowl.
- In a pan, add scallions, brown sugar, sesame oil, ginger & garlic. Cook for 15 minutes.
- Turn the heat off, add soy sauce & ketchup.
- Add the noodles & rest of the ingredients, toss & serve.

Nutrition: Kcal 460 | Protein 28 g | Fiber 9 g | Carbs 53 g | Fat 16 g

13. Slow Cooker Black Bean Soup

(Prep time: 12 hours & 15 minutes | Cook time: 11 hours |Servings: 6)

Ingredients

- 1 green bell pepper, chopped
- 3 tbsp. of fresh cilantro, chopped
- 3 garlic cloves, minced
- 1 onion, chopped
- 4 cups of vegetable broth
- 1 pound of dried black beans, rinsed
- 1 tbsp. of ground cumin
- 1 avocado, diced
- 2 tbsp. of lime juice
- 1 tsp. of salt
- 6 tsp. of light sour cream

Instructions

- Soak the beans in water for 12 hours. Drain.
- In a slow cooker, add all ingredients except for sour cream & lime juice. Cook for 10 hours on low, add lime juice.

- Pulse with a stick blender to a chunky consistency.
- Serve with sour cream on top.

Nutrition: Kcal 183 | Protein 5 g | Fiber 9 g | Carbs 29 g | Fat 4 g

14. White Bean & Avocado Sandwich

(Prep time: 15 minutes | Cook time: 0 minutes |Servings: 4)

Ingredients
- ¼ tsp. of fresh thyme, chopped
- 2 tbsp. of lemon juice
- ¼ tsp. of black pepper
- 2 avocados
- 1 tbsp. of olive oil
- 1 can of 15 oz. white beans, rinsed
- 1 cup of jarred roasted red peppers, chopped & rinsed
- 4 cups of baby lettuce
- 1 clove garlic, minced
- 8 slices of whole-wheat bread, toasted
- 8 slices of Cheddar cheese

Instructions
- In a bowl, mash the avocado with pepper, thyme, beans, oil, garlic & thyme to s chunkier consistency.
- Spread on 4 slices of bread, add cheese, red peppers & lettuce. Top with the other slice of bread.
- Slice & serve.

Nutrition: Kcal 567 | Protein 22 g | Fiber 15 g | Carbs 54 g | Fat 29 g

15. Lentil Tomato Salad

(Prep time: 15 minutes | Cook time: 0 minutes |Servings: 4)

Ingredients
- 1/4 cup of white wine vinegar
- 15 oz. of canned lentils, rinsed

- Salt, to taste
- 1 1/2 cups of cherry tomatoes, halved
- 1/8 cup of chopped chives

Instructions
- Add all ingredients to a bowl. Toss well & serve.

Nutrition: Kcal 137 | Protein 10 g | Fiber 9 g | Carbs 24 g | Fat 1 g

16. Buttermilk Bran pancakes

(Prep time: 15 minutes | Cook time: 35 minutes |Servings: 4)

Ingredients
- 2 eggs, whisked
- 1 cup of self-rising flour
- 1 tbsp. of caster sugar
- 1 tsp. of vanilla extract
- 2.1 oz. of Fiber Toppers (All-Bran)
- 1 cup of buttermilk

Poached fruit
- 7 oz. of mixed dehydrated fruit
- 1 tbsp. of caster sugar
- 1 cup of orange juice
- 1 cinnamon stick

Instructions
- In a pan, add all ingredients of poached fruits except for fruits.
- Heat on medium flame until dissolved. Boil & add fruits, simmer for 5 to 10 minutes.
- Turn the heat off & set it aside.
- In a bowl, add flour, sugar & All-Bran (half). Mix & add vanilla, eggs & buttermilk mix until smooth.
- Oil spray a pan, add batter & cook for 2-3 minutes on both sides.
- Serve with poached fruits.

Nutrition: Kcal 460 | Protein 14 g | Fiber 9 g | Carbs 23 g | Fat 6 g

17. Feta, Kale & Pear Salad

(Prep time: 15 minutes | Cook time: 15 minutes |Servings: 4)

Ingredients

- 1 tbsp. of water
- 1 ½ tsp. of olive oil
- Half tsp. of kosher salt
- ¼ cup of each pepita, sunflower seeds & sesame seeds
- ¼ cup of yogurt
- 1 ½ tsp. of cider vinegar
- ¼ red onion, sliced
- 1 tsp. of lemon juice
- 2 tbsp. of tahini
- 10 cups of torn kale leave, without stems
- Half cup of crumbled feta cheese
- 1 ripe pear, sliced
- 1 cup of fresh mint

Instructions

- Let the oven preheat to 325 F.
- Roast the seeds for 10 minutes, add to a bowl & toss with salt (1/8 tsp.) & oil.
- In a bowl, whisk yogurt with lemon juice, salt (1/8 tsp.), vinegar, tahini & water. Add kale & massage the leaves well.
- Add mint, pear & onion. Toss well.
- Serve the salad with seeds & feta.

Nutrition: Kcal 308| Protein 12 g | Fiber 8 g | Carbs 22 g | Fat 21.1 g

18. Creamy White Bean and Spinach Soup

(Prep time: 12 hours & 15 minutes | Cook time: 40 minutes |Servings: 4)

Ingredients

- 1 large onion, diced
- Half cup of dried navy beans, soaked for 12 hours
- 1 tbsp. of Dijon mustard
- 1 tbsp. of olive oil
- 2 cloves garlic, minced
- 4 cups of spinach

Instructions

- In a pot, add sauté the garlic & onion in hot olive oil for 5 minutes.
- Add water (2 cups) & beans, boil. Simmer on low for 45 minutes.
- Add mustard & spinach, pulse with a stick blender until smooth.
- Serve.

Nutrition: Kcal 98 | Protein 5 g | Fiber 7 g | Carbs 17 g | Fat 4 g

19. Bean Soup with Kale

(Prep time: 15 minutes | Cook time: 30 minutes |Servings: 4)

Ingredients

- 15 oz. of ciabatta bread
- 3 garlic cloves
- 14 oz. of canned cannellini beans, rinsed
- 1 tbsp. of olive oil
- 1 bunch of kale, without thick stems
- 14 oz. of chopped canned tomatoes with paste
- 4 cups of chicken stock

Instructions

- Let the oven preheat to 350 F.
- Toss the kale with salt & oil, bake for 10-12 minutes, flipping halfway through.
- Toast the bread slices. Rub the garlic on hot toasted bread.
- Sauté the garlic in hot oil, add stock & tomatoes. Boil & add beans, simmer for 10 minutes.
- Season with salt & pepper.

- Serve with bread & kale on top.

Nutrition: Kcal 325 | Protein 15.2 g | Fiber 10.6 g | Carbs 44 g | Fat 9.1 g

20. Ginger-Garlic Chicken Soup

(Prep time: 15 minutes | Cook time: 30 minutes |Servings: 4)

Ingredients

- Half cup of diced yellow onion
- 6 minced cloves garlic
- 3 tbsp. of oil
- 1 pound of chicken thighs, boneless, skinless, cut into half" pieces
- 4 cups of chicken broth
- 1 ½ cups of green papaya, peeled & cubed
- ¼ tsp. of salt & pepper, each
- ¼ cup of fresh ginger, sliced
- 2 cups of chopped bok choy leaves
- 1 tbsp. of fish sauce

Instructions

- Sauté garlic, onion & ginger in hot oil for 3 minutes.
- Add both & chicken, cook for 5 minutes.
- Add papaya, salt, pepper, fish sauce & bok choy. Simmer for 5 minutes.
- Serve.

Nutrition: Kcal 344| Protein 27 g | Fiber 4 g | Carbs 14 g | Fat 20 g

21. Barley with Chorizo & Tomatoes

(Prep time: 15 minutes | Cook time: 30 minutes |Servings: 4)

Ingredients

- 6 cups + ¼ cup of boiling water
- 1 tbsp. of olive oil
- 1 cup of pearl barley
- 17 oz. of chorizo, thinly sliced
- 10.5 oz. of baby brussels sprouts, halved or quartered
- 1 red onion, sliced
- 1/4 cup of chopped parsley
- Half tsp. of Paprika
- Half tsp. of ground cumin
- 8.8 oz. Roma tomatoes, halved
- 2 garlic cloves, minced

Instructions

- Add water (6 cups) & barley to a pan simmer for 25 minutes. Drain.
- In a pan, cook chorizo in oil for 2-3 minutes. Take it out on a plate.
- Add garlic, cumin, onion & paprika to a pan cook for 3 minutes.
- Add chorizo & cook for 2-3 minutes, add sprouts & cook for 3 to 4 minutes.
- Add water & cook for 2 minutes.
- Add barely & mix well. Add tomato, serve.

Nutrition: Kcal 419 | Protein 17 g | Fiber 13 g | Carbs 47 g | Fat 15 g

22. Turkey & Sweet Potato Salad

(Prep time: 15 minutes | Cook time: 0 minutes |Servings: 1)

Ingredients

- ¼ cup of chopped avocado
- Half cup of sweet potato, cooked & diced
- 3 oz. of cooked turkey, shredded
- Half oz. of Cheddar cheese, cubed
- 3 cups of chopped lettuce
- ¼ cup of sliced apple
- 2 tbsp. of apple-cider vinaigrette
- 2 tbsp. of roasted sunflower seeds

Instructions

- In a bowl, add all ingredients.
- Toss & serve.

Nutrition: Kcal 542| Protein 36 g | Fiber 10 g | Carbs 31 g | Fat 30 g

23. Charred Kale & Farro Protein Salad

(Prep time: 30 minutes | Cook time: 30 minutes |Servings: 2)

Ingredients

- 6 kale leaves, without stems & torn
- Half cup of shaved parmesan
- 1 cup of dry farro, soaked for 12 hours
- Half onion, sliced
- Salt & Pepper
- 1/4 cup of pumpkin seeds
- 2 salmon fillets

Dressing

- 1 garlic clove, minced
- 2 tbsp. of each olive oil & lemon juice
- 1/4 tsp. of each salt & pepper

Instructions

- In a pan, add soaked farro add enough water to cover it.
- Boil & simmer for 20 minutes.
- Let the oven preheat to 425 F.
- Coat the salmon in oil season with salt & pepper.
- Bake for 6 to 10 minutes.
- In a pan, add a drizzle of oil. Sauté kale for 2-3 minutes until charred.
- Take it out on a plate, add onion & char them.
- Toss all of the ingredients except for salmon. Serve with salmon.

Nutrition: Kcal 301| Protein 11 g | Fiber 10 g | Carbs 13 g | Fat 7 g

24. Charred Broccoli Salad with Arugula

(Prep time: 15 minutes | Cook time: 10 minutes |Servings: 4-6)

Ingredients

- 3 tbsp. of olive oil
- 1 anchovy fillet, oil-packed
- 2 garlic cloves
- 1 1/2 tsp. of Dijon mustard
- 2/3 cup of mayonnaise
- 2 heads of broccoli, broken into florets
- 1/4 cup of chopped chives
- 1/4 cup of buttermilk
- 1 cup of parsley
- 1 cup of tarragon leaves
- 3.5 oz. of smoked cheddar, shaved
- 1 lemon's juice
- 4 cups of baby arugula
- Salt & pepper

Instructions

- Boil broccoli for 2 minutes in salted water until tender.
- Add to cold water & drain. Add to a skillet sauté in hot oil for 5-10 minutes.
- Sprinkle salt on top.
- Add the rest of the ingredients to a bowl except for arugula. Whisk well
- Add broccoli & arugula. Toss & serve.

Nutrition: Kcal 265| Protein 4 g | Fiber 10 g | Carbs 7 g | Fat 6 g

25. Lemon Chicken Orzo Soup

(Prep time: 15 minutes | Cook time: 10 minutes |Servings: 6)

Ingredients

- 1 pound of chicken breasts, boneless & skinless, cubed
- 1 tsp. of dried oregano
- 1 ¼ tsp. of salt
- 4 cups of chicken broth
- 2 tbsp. of olive oil
- ⅔ cup of orzo pasta
- 2 cups of chopped onions
- 1 cup of chopped carrots
- ¾ tsp. of black pepper
- 1 lemon, zest & juice
- 1 cup chopped celery
- 2 cloves garlic, minced

- 1 bay leaf
- 4 cups of chopped kale

Instructions

- Cook chicken in oil (1 tbsp.) with oregano (half), salt & pepper for 3-5 minutes.
- Take it out on a plate.
- Add the oil & sauté celery, onion & carrots for 3-5 minutes. Add half oregano, garlic & bay leaf. Cook for 30-60 seconds.
- Add broth, boil & add orzo. Simmer for 5 minutes.
- Add chicken & kale, cook for 5-8 minutes.
- Turn the heat off, take the bay leaf out.
- Add the rest of the ingredients. Serve.

Nutrition: Kcal 245 | Protein 21.1 g | Fiber 6 g | Carbs 24 g | Fat 7 g

26. Southwestern Chopped Salad

(Prep time: 15 minutes | Cook time: 0 minutes |Servings: 1)

Ingredients

For Dressing

- 1/4 cup of yogurt
- Half cup of Red Enchilada Sauce

For Salad

- 1 cup of shredded purple cabbage
- Half cup of cooked freekeh
- Half cup of canned black beans, rinsed
- 2 tbsp. of chopped green onions
- 1/4 cup of chopped red bell peppers
- 1 Roma tomato, diced without seeds
- 3 tbsp. of dressing
- Half cup of diced jicama
- Half cup of sweet corn
- Cilantro, to taste

Instructions

- Whisk the dressing ingredients.
- In a mason jar, add the salad's ingredients, shake well & serve.

Nutrition: Kcal 426 | Protein 21 g | Fiber 1.2 g | Carbs 89 g | Fat 2.5 g

27. Black Bean & Barley Cakes

(Prep time: 15 minutes | Cook time: 20 minutes |Servings: 4)

Ingredients

- 1 oz. of porridge oats
- 2 tsp. of thyme leaves
- 2 tsp. of ground coriander
- 2 cans of (14 oz.) black beans, drained
- 1 tsp. of cumin seeds
- 5 eggs
- 7 oz. of cherry tomatoes
- 2 scallions, sliced
- 1 tsp. of vegetable bouillon
- 17 oz. of canned barley, drained
- 4 tbsp. of sunflower seeds
- 2-3 tsp. of rapeseed oil

Instructions

- In a food processor, add cumin seeds, bouillon powder, oats, thyme, beans & ground coriander. Pulse into a paste.
- Mix with one egg white with barley & scallions.
- In a pan, add oil add the mixture with a spoon & make cakes. Cook for 7 minutes & 4-5 minutes on the other side.
- Poach the eggs, fry the tomatoes.
- Serve the cakes with eggs & tomatoes.

Nutrition: Kcal 343 | Protein 20 g | Fiber 10 g | Carbs 26 g | Fat 15 g

28. Posh Beans On Toast

(Prep time: 15 minutes | Cook time: 1 hour & 20 minutes |Servings: 4)

Ingredients

- 3/4 cup of olive oil
- 1 tbsp. of wholegrain mustard
- 5 garlic cloves, diced
- 8.8 oz. of dried cannellini beans, soaked overnight
- 1 onion, chopped
- 2 tsp. of chopped thyme leaves
- Half cup of parsley leaves
- 14 oz. of canned chopped tomatoes
- 2 tbsp. of sun-dried tomato paste
- 1/4 cup of each brown sugar & cider vinegar
- 2 tbsp. of curry powder
- 21 oz. of Tomato Passata
- 21 oz. of chicken stock

Instructions

- Simmer the beans & water for 45 minutes.
- In a pan, add half a cup of oil with thyme, garlic & onion; cook for 2-3 minutes.
- Add the drained beans with the rest of the ingredients except for oil & parsley.
- Cook for 45 minutes. Adjust seasoning.
- Heat the oil in a pan fry parsley leaves for 20 seconds.
- Serve beans with fried leaves & toast.

Nutrition: Kcal 289 | Protein 9 g | Fiber 10 g | Carbs 15 g | Fat 6 g

29. Healthy Chopped Salad

(Prep time: 15 minutes | Cook time: 0 minutes |Servings: 4)

Ingredients

- 1 cup of cooked chicken breast, shredded
- 1/4 cup of goat cheese, crumbled
- 1 can of (15.5 oz.) chickpeas, rinsed
- 2 romaine hearts, chopped
- 1 cup of grape tomatoes, halved
- Half cup of BBQ dressing
- 3/4 cup of sweet corn
- 1/3 cup of cilantro
- 1 avocado, diced

Instructions

- Add all ingredients to a bowl, except for dressing & avocado.
- Toss & serve with dressing & avocado.

Nutrition: Kcal 257 | Protein 11 g | Fiber 9.8 g | Carbs 7 g | Fat 5 g

30. Quinoa Black Bean Salad

(Prep time: 15 minutes | Cook time: 30 minutes |Servings: 6)

Ingredients

- 1 red onion cut, largely chopped
- 3 tbsp. of lime juice
- 1 clove garlic, minced
- 1 1/4 pounds of peeled sweet potatoes, largely cubed
- 1 tsp. of smoked paprika
- Half tsp. of kosher salt
- 1 1/2 cups of cooked quinoa
- 4 tbsp. of olive oil
- Zest of 2 limes
- 3/4 cup of cilantro
- 2 tsp. of maple syrup
- 1 can of (15 oz.) black beans, rinsed
- 1 bell pepper, diced

Instructions

- Let the oven preheat to 400 F.
- Toss the potatoes & onion in oil (1tbsp.), salt & paprika and bake for 25 minutes.

- In a bowl, whisk the oil (3 tbsp.), garlic, lime juice, maple syrup & zest.
- Add the rest of the ingredients to a bowl, add dressing, toss & serve.

Nutrition: Kcal 312 | Protein 8 g | Fiber 23 g | Carbs 49 g | Fat 11 g

6.3 DINNER

1. Lentil Fritters

(Prep time: 15 minutes | Cook time: 10 minutes |Servings: 2)

Ingredients

- ½ cup of chopped coriander
- 1 sliced scallion
- ½ tsp. of sesame seeds
- 1.7 oz. of gram flour
- 10.5 oz. of cooked basic lentils
- 1 tbsp. of rapeseed oil
- 2 carrots
- ½ tsp. of sesame oil
- 2 courgettes
- 1 lime's juice

Instructions

- Cut the courgettes & carrots into ribbons & mix with lime juice, sesame oil & coriander.
- Mix the lentils with flour & scallion. Let it rest for a few minutes.
- In a pan, heat the oil. Add the spoonful of lentil mixture & make it into cakes.
- Serve with ribbon sides.

Nutrition: Kcal 356 | Protein 0.1 g | Fiber 11 g | Carbs 41 g | Fat 12 g

2. Curried Quinoa Wraps

(Prep time: 15 minutes | Cook time: 0 minutes |Servings: 2)

Ingredients

- ½ cup of pumpkin puree
- 1 tsp. of paprika
- 1 cup of alfalfa sprouts
- 1 cucumber, cut into ribbons
- 1 tsp. of curry powder
- Salt, to taste
- 12 small collard leaves
- 1 cup of cooked quinoa
- 1 avocado, sliced thin

Sauce

- 1 tbsp. of lime juice
- 2 tbsp. of tahini
- 1 tbsp. of olive oil

Instructions

- In a bowl, mix curry powder, quinoa, salt, pumpkin puree, paprika & salt, mix well.
- Take the stems out of the leaves & add some of the fillings in each leaf.
- Add ribbons, sprouts & avocado.
- Whisk the seasoning & drizzle in each of the wraps.

Nutrition: Kcal 470 | Protein 10 g | Fiber 13 g | Carbs 41 g | Fat 32 g

3. Turkey Tortilla Wrap

(Prep time: 15 minutes | Cook time: 0 minutes |Servings: 2)

Ingredients

- 2 to 3 tbsp. of Greek yogurt
- 2 tsp. of lemon juice
- ½ avocado
- 4 oz. of sliced turkey
- 2 spinach leaves
- Salt and pepper, to taste
- 2 whole-grain tortillas
- 1 large Roma tomato, sliced thin

Instructions

- In a food processor, pulse the avocado, pepper, yogurt, salt & lemon juice. Pulse until smooth.
- Place one tortilla and add some of the yogurt creams with the rest of the ingredients on top.
- Roll & slice. Serve.

Nutrition: Kcal 89 | Protein 8 g | Fiber 8.9 g | Carbs 12 g | Fat 4.2 g

4. Chorizo & Pinto Bean Chili

(Prep time: 15 minutes | Cook time: 35 minutes |Servings: 4)

Ingredients

- 12 oz. of chorizo, without casing
- 1 yellow onion, diced
- 1 tsp. of kosher salt
- 1 tsp. of garlic powder
- 1 poblano chili, chopped without stem (optional)
- 1 tbsp. of olive oil
- 1 tbsp. of tomato paste
- 3 cups of chicken broth
- 1 tsp. of ground cumin
- 2 cans of (15 oz.) pinto beans, rinsed

Instructions

- Brown the chorizo for 2-3 minutes. Drain all but one tbsp. of fat & take the chorizo out on a plate.
- Add chili & onion to a pot cook for 5 minutes.
- Add seasonings & cook for 1 minute.
- Mash one cup of beans & add to the pot with all the ingredients.
- Simmer for 5 minutes. Serve.

Nutrition: Kcal 606 | Protein 26 g | Fiber 10 g | Carbs 41 g | Fat 39 g

5. Beef and Lentil Stew

(Prep time: 15 minutes | Cook time: 1 hour & 20 minutes |Servings: 8)

Ingredients

- 2 ½ pounds of beef chuck, cubed
- 1 onion, chopped
- 3 celery stalks, sliced
- 3 garlic cloves, minced
- 2 tbsp. of olive oil
- 4 carrots, sliced
- Salt & Pepper, to taste
- 3 tbsp. of fresh tarragon, chopped
- 1 ½ cup of dried lentils, brown
- 1 cup of dry red wine
- 28 oz. of canned crushed tomatoes
- 6 cups of beef stock
- 3 bay leaves
- 1 tbsp. of dried thyme
- Cayenne pepper, a pinch

Instructions

- Sauté the onion, garlic & beef in hot oil for 5-10 minutes.
- Add the rest of the ingredients.
- Let it come to a boil, turn the heat low and simmer for 1 hour & 5-10 minutes more.
- Adjust seasoning & serve.

Nutrition: Kcal 524 | Protein 42 g | Fiber 14 g | Carbs 38 g | Fat 7 g

6. Pea & Spinach Carbonara

(Prep time: 15 minutes | Cook time: 25 minutes |Servings: 4)

Ingredients

- ½ cup of whole-wheat panko
- 1 minced clove garlic
- ½ tsp. of pepper
- 8 tbsp. of grated Parmesan
- 1 cup of peas
- 1 ½ tbsp. of olive oil
- 3 tbsp. of parsley
- 3 egg yolks
- 8 cups of baby spinach
- 1 egg
- ¼ tsp. of salt
- 1 pack of (9 oz.) linguine

Instructions

- Heat oil in a pan, add garlic & breadcrumbs, cook for 2 minutes.

Take it out in a bowl & mix with parmesan (2 tbsp.).

- In a bowl, whisk yolk with salt, egg, parmesan, pepper.
- Cook pasta as per package instructions, at the last one minute.
- Add peas & spinach, drain all but ¼ cup of water.
- Add ¼ cup of water to the egg mixture.
- Add to the pasta mixture, mix well. Serve with breadcrumbs.

Nutrition: Kcal 430 | Protein 20 g | Fiber 9 g | Carbs 54 g | Fat 14 g

7. Pork Sausage & Green Lentil Braise

(Prep time: 15 minutes | Cook time: 25 minutes |Servings: 6)

Ingredients

- 1.4 oz. of butter
- 2 thyme sprigs
- 2 onions, chopped
- 3 garlic cloves, minced
- 1 tbsp. of olive oil
- 2 bacon rashers, chopped
- 1 carrot, chopped
- 6 thick pork sausages
- 2 celery stalks, chopped
- 2 cups of red wine
- 14 oz. of 2 cans green lentils, rinsed

Instructions

- Sauté bacon, onion & garlic for 4-6 minutes in butter (half).
- Add celery & carrot, cook for 8 to 10 minutes.
- Add red wine simmer for 6 to 8 minutes.
- Add lentils & thyme, simmer for half an hour. Add the rest of the butter.

- Grill sausages for 6-8 minutes, serve with lentils.

Nutrition: Kcal 289 | Protein 5 g | Fiber 12 g | Carbs 15 g | Fat 5 g

8. Lentils & Crispy Brussel Sprouts

(Prep time: 15 minutes | Cook time: 35 minutes |Servings: 6)

Ingredients

- 2 shallots, cut into wedges
- 2 ½ tbsp. of olive oil
- 1 garlic clove, sliced
- 4 large Portobello mushrooms
- ½ cup of dried puy lentils washed
- 8 oz. Brussels sprouts halved
- 0.8 oz. butter, chopped
- 1 tsp. of thyme leaves
- 2 tbsp. of cider vinegar
- ½ cup of pecans halved
- 1 radicchio, torn leaves
- 2 tbsp. of fresh parsley, chopped

Instructions

- Let the oven preheat to 400°F.
- Toss the shallots & sprouts with salt, pepper & oil (1 tbsp.).
- Toss the mushrooms with salt, thyme, pepper & oil (1 tbsp.).
- Place on two different baking trays.
- Roast for 25 minutes. Cook lentils as per package instructions.
- Toast pecans in the rest of the oil, add garlic & radicchio. Cook for 3-4 minutes.
- Add lentils, shallots & sprouts. Add vinegar, salt, pepper & parsley.
- Toss & serve with mushrooms.

Nutrition: Kcal 373 | Protein 11.8 g | Fiber 12.2 g | Carbs 11 g | Fat 27 g

9. Bean & Spinach Enchiladas

(Prep time: 15 minutes | Cook time: 3 hours & 35 minutes | Servings: 6)

Ingredients

- 10 oz. of squeezed thawed spinach
- 1 cup of corn
- ½ tsp. of ground cumin
- 8 oz. of sharp Cheddar, grated
- ½ cup of grape tomatoes halved
- 8 corn (6") tortillas, warmed
- 1 can of (~16 oz.) black beans, rinsed
- Salt & black pepper
- 3 ½ cups of jarred salsa
- 6 cups of chopped romaine lettuce
- 4 radishes, sliced thin
- 2 tbsp. of olive oil
- ½ cucumber, sliced
- 3 tbsp. of lime juice

Instructions

- Mash beans (only half) mix with cheddar (1 cup), corn, rest of the beans, salt, spinach, pepper & cumin.
- In a slow cooker (4-6 qt.), spread one salsa jar.
- In each tortilla, fill the bean mixture & roll.
- Place in the slow cooker. Add cheddar & all the salsa on top.
- Cook for 2 ½-3 hours.
- Add the rest of the ingredients to a bowl, with salt & pepper, toss & serve with rolls.

Nutrition: Kcal 576 | Protein 28 g | Fiber 12 g | Carbs 60 g | Fat 28 g

10. Lentil Quinoa Meatballs

(Prep time: 15 minutes | Cook time: 60 minutes | Servings: 8)

Ingredients

- ¼ cup of uncooked quinoa
- 1 tbsp. of ground flaxseed
- 5 oz. of cremini mushrooms
- 3 cups of water
- 1 cup of chopped red onion
- ¾ cup of uncooked french lentils
- 1 cup of rolled oats
- 3 tbsp. of water
- ¼ cup of sunflower seeds ground
- 2 tbsp. of tomato paste
- 2 tbsp. of nutritional yeast
- 1 tsp. of dried parsley
- 2 garlic cloves, minced
- 1 tbsp. of Worcestershire sauce
- ¼ tsp. of black pepper
- 1 tbsp. of Italian seasonings
- 1 tsp. of dried basil
- ½ tsp. of sea salt

Instructions

- Rinse & drain the lentils & quinoa.
- Boil 3 cups of water with salt & add lentils; cook for 24 minutes.
- After 12 minutes, add the quinoa & cook for 12 minutes more or until liquid is absorbed.
- In a bowl, add water (3 tbsp.) & ground flaxseed (1 tbsp.), keep in the fridge for 10 minutes.
- Grind the seeds into powder.
- Add the lentil mixture to a food processor with all of the ingredients.
- Pulse for 1 to 2 minutes until sticky. Make into balls & place on parchment-lined baking sheets.
- Let the oven preheat to 350°F.
- Bake for 15 to 18 minutes.

Nutrition: Kcal 360 | Protein 20 g | Fiber 18 g | Carbs 55 g | Fat 8 g

11. Beef & Bean Sloppy Joes

(Prep time: 15 minutes | Cook time: 30 minutes |Servings: 4)

Ingredients

- 12 oz. of ground beef
- 2 tsp. of spicy brown mustard
- 1 cup of canned black beans, rinsed
- 1 cup of diced onion
- ½ tsp. of each garlic powder & onion powder
- 1 cup of tomato sauce
- 1 tbsp. of olive oil
- 4 hamburger buns, whole-wheat, halved & toasted
- 3 tbsp. of ketchup
- 1 tbsp. of Worcestershire sauce
- 1 tsp. of light brown sugar

Instructions

- Cook the beef in hot oil for 3-5 minutes & take it on a plate.
- Add onion & beans, cook for 5 minutes.
- Add seasoning cook for 30 seconds.
- Add the rest of the ingredients with beef cook for 5 minutes.
- Serve on toasted buns

Nutrition: Kcal 411 | Protein 25 g | Fiber 9 g | Carbs 43 g | Fat 15 g

12. Lamb with Lentils, Feta & Mint

(Prep time: 15 minutes | Cook time: 30 minutes |Servings: 4)

Ingredients

- 1/4 cup of olive oil
- ½ cup of Kalamata olives, chopped
- 1 tbsp. of lemon juice
- 5 oz. of feta, crumbled
- 7 oz. of 2 lamb back straps, trimmed
- 9 oz. of cherry tomatoes
- 1 tbsp. of chopped rosemary
- 2 tbsp. of mint leaves
- 14 oz. of canned lentils, rinsed
- 1 tsp. of dried mint

Instructions

- Let the oven preheat to 400 F.
- Coat the tomatoes in oil (2 tsp.), roast for 15 minutes, after 10 minutes, add olives.
- Season the lamb with salt, pepper, oil (2 tsp.) & rosemary. Brown in the pan for 3 minutes on each side.
- Cover them in foil loosely.
- Simmer the lentils in water for 5 minutes, drain & toss with oil (2 tbsp.), salt, pepper & lemon juice.
- Serve the lamb with lentils & the rest of the ingredients.

Nutrition: Kcal 301| Protein 14 g | Fiber 9 g | Carbs 13 g | Fat 6 g

13. Bean Chili

(Prep time: 15 minutes | Cook time: 30 minutes |Servings: 4)

Ingredients

- 1 onion, chopped
- 14 oz. of the canned mixed bean, rinsed
- 1 tbsp. of sunflower oil
- 2 cans of (14 oz.) black beans, rinsed
- 1 tbsp. of brown sugar
- 4 eggs
- 2 cans of (14 oz.) chopped tomatoes with herbs & garlic

Instructions

- Sauté onion in hot oil for 5 minutes.
- Add the rest of the ingredients, except for eggs, simmer for 15 to 20 minutes.
- Make four holes & add one egg in each hole. Simmer for 8-10 minutes.

- Serve.

Nutrition: Kcal 377 | Protein 24 g | Fiber 15 g | Carbs 48 g | Fat 10 g

14. Mexican Quinoa Wraps

(Prep time: 15 minutes | Cook time: 10 minutes |Servings: 6)

Ingredients

- 1 onion, chopped
- 1 cup of uncooked quinoa
- 15 oz. of canned black beans
- 1 red pepper, chopped
- 7 oz. of canned corn

Instructions

- Cook quinoa. Chop the vegetables.
- Sauté the vegetables in hot oil for 5 minutes.
- In each tortilla, add some of the ingredients. Roll & serve.

Nutrition: Kcal 543 | Protein 15 g | Fiber 8 g | Carbs 18.7 g | Fat 22 g

15. Grilled Chicken Wrap

(Prep time: 15 minutes | Cook time: 8 minutes |Servings: 6)

Ingredients

- 1 tbsp. of olive oil
- 1 cucumber, diced
- 6 Tortilla Wraps (Whole Wheat)
- 1 ¼ - 1 ½ pound of Chicken Tenders
- 8 oz. of Roasted Garlic Hummus
- Feta cheese, crumbled
- Baby Spinach, as needed
- Grape Tomatoes, chopped

Spice Blend

- ½ tsp. of each oregano & paprika
- ⅛ tsp. of garlic powder
- ¼ tsp. of each cumin & sea salt

Instructions

- Let the grill preheat to medium.

- Season the chicken with the spice blend. Grill the chicken until done
- On every tortilla, spread the hummus. Add the chicken with the rest of the ingredients.
- Roll & serve.

Nutrition: Kcal 234 | Protein 8.9 g | Fiber 10.2 g | Carbs 12 g | Fat 5 g

16. Teriyaki Tofu Rice Bowls

(Prep time: 15 minutes | Cook time: 8 minutes |Servings: 4)

Ingredients

- 1 tbsp. of olive oil
- 1 pack of (7 oz.) teriyaki-flavor baked tofu, cut into cubes
- 1 pack of (18 oz.) stir-fry vegetables
- 2 packs of (10 oz.) frozen wild rice
- 3 tbsp. of teriyaki sauce

Instructions

- Cook rice as per package instructions.
- Sauté vegetables in hot oil for 4-5 minutes with sauce.
- Serve the rice with vegetables & tofu.

Nutrition: Kcal 360 | Protein 15.2 g | Fiber 9 g | Carbs 59 g | Fat 8 g

17. Salmon with Spinach Rice

(Prep time: 15 minutes | Cook time: 20 minutes |Servings: 4)

Ingredients

- 1-inch piece of ginger, peeled & grated
- 1/4 cup of tamari
- 2 garlic cloves, minced
- 1 tbsp. mirin
- 1 tsp. Wasabi paste
- 1 tsp. of caster sugar
- 2 tsp. of sesame seeds
- 1 cup of Rice & Quinoa

- 4 cups of frozen edamame, thawed
- 3.5 oz. snow peas halved
- 1.7 oz. baby spinach
- 2 tsp. of sesame oil
- 3 scallions, sliced
- 4 salmon fillets, skinless & boneless

Instructions
- Let the oven preheat to 400°F.
- Add all ingredients in a bowl, except for rice, spinach, snow peas, soybeans & fish.
- In each foil paper, add parchment paper, place fish & drizzle sauce on top. Coat & wrap, bake for 20 minutes.
- Cook rice as per package instructions, add soybeans in the last five minutes.
- Add the sauce with oil, toss & add spinach. Let it rest for 5 minutes.
- Serve with fish.

Nutrition: Kcal 563 | Protein 40 g | Fiber 6 g | Carbs 46 g | Fat 22 g

18. Cauliflower and Chickpea Stew

(Prep time: 15 minutes | Cook time: 8 minutes |Servings: 4)
Ingredients
- 1 onion, diced
- 1 can of 28 oz. whole tomatoes
- 1 ½ tsp. of ground cumin
- 2 tbsp. of olive oil
- Half tsp. of ground ginger
- Half cup of raisins
- Salt & black pepper
- 1 can of 15 oz. chickpeas, rinsed
- 1 cup of couscous
- 1 head of cauliflower, broken into florets
- 1 pack of 5 oz. baby spinach, chopped

Instructions
- Sauté the onion in hot oil for 4-5 minutes.
- Add salt, pepper, ginger & cumin, cook for 1 minute.
- Add water (half cup) with tomatoes, chickpeas, raisins & cauliflower.
- Let it come to a boil, turn the heat low and simmer for 15-20 minutes.
- Add spinach & cook for 1-2 minutes.
- Cook quinoa & serve with stew.

Nutrition: Kcal 446| Protein 16 g | Fiber 13 g | Carbs 18.7 g | Fat 9 g

19. Bean & Meat Loaf

(Prep time: 15 minutes | Cook time: 1 hour & 40 minutes |Servings: 4)
Ingredients
- 3/4 cup of a kidney bean, cooked
- 1 tbsp. of Italian herb seasoning
- ½ tsp. of black pepper
- 2 eggs
- 1 tbsp. of tamari
- 1/3 cup of rolled oats
- 2 tbsp. of dried onion flakes
- ½ cup of bell pepper, minced
- 15 oz. of ground beef
- 1 cup of tomato sauce
- ½ cup of celery, minced
- 3/4 tsp. of garlic powder

Instructions
- Let the oven preheat to 350°F.
- Blend the eggs with tamari, beans, pepper & herb blend.
- Add the rest of the ingredients to the bean mixture except for a half cup of tomato sauce.
- Oil spray a loaf pan, add the mixture and top with tomato sauce.
- Bake for 1-1 ¼ hours.

Nutrition: Kcal 234 | Protein 15 g | Fiber 8.9 g | Carbs 13 g | Fat 8 g

20. Southwest Chicken

(Prep time: 15 minutes | Cook time: 40 minutes |Servings: 4)

Ingredients

- 4 chicken breast halves, skinless & boneless
- 1 can of 9 oz. kernel corn, drained
- 1 pinch of ground cumin
- 1 can of 10 oz. diced tomatoes
- 1 tbsp. of vegetable oil
- 1 can of 15 oz. black beans, rinsed

Instructions

- Cook chicken in hot oil until browned.
- Add the corn, tomatoes & beans. Simmer for half an hour.
- Serve with cumin.

Nutrition: Kcal 310 | Protein 35 g | Fiber 7.5 g | Carbs 27 g | Fat 6 g

21. Beef & Broccoli Stir-fry

(Prep time: 15 minutes | Cook time: 15 minutes |Servings: 2)

Ingredients

- 2 cups of broccoli, diced
- 1 tsp. of salt
- 1 lb. of flank steak, cubed
- 1 tsp. of pepper

Sauce

- 1 tbsp. of sesame seed
- ¼ cup of honey
- ½ cup of soy sauce
- 2 cloves of garlic
- 1 tsp. of ginger

Instructions

- Add all ingredients of sauce in a bowl & mix.
- Cook beef in hot oil until browned.

- Add sauce, cook for 2 minutes, add vegetables. Cook until tender.
- Serve.

Nutrition: Kcal 715 | Protein 72 g | Fiber 7 g | Carbs 20 g | Fat 22 g

22. Prosciutto Pizza with Corn & Arugula

(Prep time: 15 minutes | Cook time: 40 minutes |Servings: 4)

Ingredients

- 2 tbsp. of olive oil, divided
- 1 clove garlic, minced
- 1 oz. of sliced prosciutto, torn
- 1 cup of mozzarella cheese, shredded
- 1 pound of whole-wheat pizza dough
- ¼ tsp. of ground pepper
- 1 cup of fresh corn
- 1 ½ cups of arugula
- ½ cup of torn fresh basil

Instructions

- Let the grill preheat to medium.
- Roll the dough. Mix the garlic with 1 tbsp. of oil.
- Oil spray the grill & grill the dough for 1-2 minutes.
- Flip & spread garlic oil, add corn, cheese & prosciutto.
- Grill for 2-3 minutes. Add the rest of the ingredients,
- Slice & serve.

Nutrition: Kcal 436 | Protein 18 g | Fiber 4 g | Carbs 53 g | Fat 19 g

23. Moroccan Lamb & Lentil Soup

(Prep time: 15 minutes | Cook time: 2 hours |Servings: 6)

Ingredients

- 24 oz. of diced lamb
- 1 onion, chopped
- 2 tsp. of sweet paprika

- 2 tbsp. of olive oil
- 2 tbsp. of tomato paste
- 2 (14 oz.) cans Thick Tomatoes
- 2 garlic cloves, minced
- 11/2 tsp. of ground cumin
- Half tsp. of ground cloves
- 1 bay leaf
- 2 (14 oz.) cans chickpeas, rinsed
- 4 cups of beef stock
- 2 (14 oz.) cans brown lentils, rinsed
- ½ bunch of coriander, chopped

Instructions

- Season the lamb & cook for 4 to 5 minutes in hot oil; take it out on a plate.
- Sauté garlic & onion for 3 to 4 minutes.
- Add lamb, spices, bay leaf & tomato paste. Cook for 1 minute.
- Add coriander, tomatoes & stock. Simmer for 60 minutes.
- Add lentils & chickpeas, cook for half an hour.
- Serve.

Nutrition: Kcal 376 | Protein 13 g | Fiber 9 g | Carbs 18 g | Fat 07 g

24. Prosciutto, Kale & Bean Stew

(Prep time: 15 minutes | Cook time: 30 minutes |Servings: 4)

Ingredients

- 2 tbsp. of olive oil
- 1 fennel bulb, sliced
- 5 oz. of chicken stock
- 4 thyme sprigs
- 2.8 oz. prosciutto, torn
- 1 can of (14 oz.) cherry tomatoes
- 2 garlic clove, minced
- 2 cans of (14 oz.) butter beans
- 7 oz. of sliced kale

Instructions

- Sauté the prosciutto in a pan until crispy. Take half of it out.
- Add oil, salt & fennel. Cook for 5 minutes.
- Add thyme & garlic cook for 2 minutes.
- Add stock & simmer.
- Add all cans & simmer for 15 minutes. Add kale & cook for 1-2 minutes.
- Serve with crispy prosciutto.

Nutrition: Kcal 290| Protein 16 g | Fiber 12 g | Carbs 23 g | Fat 9 g

25. Mustardy Salmon with Lentils & Beetroot

(Prep time: 15 minutes | Cook time: 30 minutes |Servings: 2)

Ingredients

- 1 tsp. of wholegrain mustard
- ½ tsp. of honey
- 2 tbsp. of olive oil
- 2 salmon fillets
- 1 small pack of dill, chopped
- 8.8 oz. cooked puy lentils
- 2 tbsp. toasted pumpkin seeds
- 8.8 oz. cooked beetroot, cut into wedges
- 2 tbsp. of crème fraîche
- 1-2 tbsp. of capers
- ½ lemon, zest & wedged

Instructions

- Let the oven preheat to 400°F.
- Mix seasonings, mustard & oil (1 tbsp.). Spread all over the fish.
- In a dish, add the beetroot & lentils, add the rest of the oil & seasonings.
- Bake the fish & lentil mixture for 10 minutes.
- Add the rest of the ingredients to the lentil mixture.

- Serve with salmon.

Nutrition: Kcal 875 | Protein 58 g | Fiber 15 g | Carbs 42 g | Fat 49 g

26. Greek Quinoa Bowls

(Prep time: 15 minutes | Cook time: 15 minutes |Servings: 3)

Ingredients

- 1.5 cups of water
- 2 to 3 tbsp. of apple cider vinegar
- 1 cup of quinoa
- 1 cup of diced green bell pepper
- 1-2 tbsp. of fresh parsley
- 1/3 cup of feta cheese, crumbled
- 1/4 cup of olive oil
- 1 cup of diced red bell pepper
- Salt and pepper to taste
- Light dressing, as needed

Instructions

- Cook quinoa as per package instructions.
- Chop the vegetables & sauté with seasoning.
- Serve the quinoa with vegetables & dressing.

Nutrition: Kcal 440 | Protein 11 g | Fiber 7 g | Carbs 20 g | Fat 5 g

27. Falafel Tabbouleh Bowls

(Prep time: 15 minutes | Cook time: 5 minutes |Servings: 4)

Ingredients

- 1 pack of 12 oz. frozen falafel
- 7 oz. of tabbouleh
- ½ cup of tzatziki sauce
- 5 oz. of salad greens

Instructions

- Prepare the ingredients.
- In four serving bowls, divide the ingredients.

- Serve.

Nutrition: Kcal 416 | Protein 10 g | Fiber 8 g | Carbs 37 g | Fat 25 g

28. Garlic Roasted Salmon

(Prep time: 15 minutes | Cook time: 15 minutes |Servings: 6)

Ingredients

- Salt & pepper, to taste
- 1 tbsp. of Garlic Oil
- 2 pounds of salmon fillet, cut into 6 pieces
- 3-4 garlic cloves, minced
- 1 tbsp. of dried oregano

Instructions

- Let the oven preheat to 450°F.
- Oil spray a baking sheet.
- Coat salmon in garlic oil. Add pressed garlic on top & season with salt, oregano & pepper.
- Bake for 10-12 minutes, serve with rice.

Nutrition: Kcal 300 | Protein 35 g | Fiber 6 g | Carbs 14 g | Fat 19 g

29. Zucchini-Chickpea Veggie Burgers

(Prep time: 15 minutes | Cook time: 10 minutes |Servings: 4)

Ingredients

- 1 ¼ tsp. of garlic powder
- 3 tsp. of white miso
- 4 tbsp. of tahini
- 1 ¼ tsp. of black pepper
- 2 tsp. of chopped fresh chives
- 1 tbsp. of lemon juice
- ¼ cup of fresh parsley
- 1 can of 15 oz. chickpeas, rinsed
- 4 whole-grain toasted hamburger buns

- 4 slices of tomato
- 1 ¼ tsp. of onion powder
- 2 tbsp. of water
- 1 tsp. of ground cumin
- 1 tbsp. of olive oil
- ¼ tsp. of salt
- Half cup of shredded zucchini
- ⅓ cup of rolled oats
- 1 cup of fresh arugula

Instructions

- In a bowl, whisk tahini (2 tbsp.), onion powder (half tsp.), lemon juice, black pepper (1/4 tsp.), miso (1 tsp.), chives (half), garlic powder (1/4 tsp.), little water, until it is smooth.
- In a food processor, add chickpeas with onion powder, tahini, miso, pepper, garlic powder, salt & cumin. Pulse until it is smooth.
- Mix with chives & parsley.
- Squeeze the zucchini. Add to the chickpeas with oats. Mix & make into patties.
- Cook the patties in hot oil for 4-5 minutes. Flip & cook for 2-4 minutes.
- Serve with sauce in buns with tomato & arugula.

Nutrition: Kcal 373 | Protein 12 g | Fiber 10 g | Carbs 48 g | Fat 14 g

30. Pork Sausages with Cider Lentils

(Prep time: 15 minutes | Cook time: 50 minutes |Servings: 4)

Ingredients

- 2 tbsp. of olive oil
- 8 thick pork sausages
- 1 small bunch of thyme
- 2 onions, diced
- 2 cups of green lentils, rinsed
- 1 1/3 cups of Chicken Stock
- 3 garlic cloves, minced
- 1 apple, peeled & cubed
- 1 bay leaf
- 1 1/3 cups of alcoholic apple cider

Instructions

- Cook lentils for 15 to 20 minutes in boiling water, drain.
- Cook sausages in hot oil for 6 to 8 minutes. Take it out on a plate.
- Sauté garlic & onion in hot oil for 2-3 minutes.
- Add seasoning, thyme, bay leaf & apple, cook for 3-4 minutes.
- Add stock cider cook for 7 to 8 minutes.
- Add the sausage back to the pan cook for 4 to 5 minutes.
- Serve.

Nutrition: Kcal 287 | Protein 8 g | Fiber 12 g | Carbs 12 g | Fat 7 g

CHAPTER 7: 60-DAY MEAL PLAN

In this comprehensive book, we reveal the transformative power of having a meal plan at your fingertips. With a meal plan, you can effortlessly improve your diet and overall health. Say hello to balanced nutrition, controlled portions, and the freedom to choose the foods you love while staying on track with your wellness goals. Our carefully crafted meal plans take the guesswork out of your daily menu, allowing you to savor your meals with peace of mind.

WEEK 1 : CLEAR DIET PHASE

The Calming Phase: Ease inflammation during a flare-up by following a low-residue, low-fiber diet. Focus on broths, cooked refined grains, ripe bananas, and tender cooked vegetables/proteins to allow intestinal healing.

DAYS	BREAKFAST	LUNCH	DINNER
MON	Apple juice, 4.1.1	Peach Iced Tea, 4.1.7	Chicken Clear Soup, 4.2.3
TUE	Smooth Sweet Tea, 4.1.2	Clear vegetable soup, 4.2.2	Garlic Chicken Soup, 4.2.5
WED	Lemon Ginger Detox Tea, 4.1.10	Basic Bone Broth, 4.2.1	Easy Miso Soup, 4.2.8
THU	Warm Honey Green Tea, 4.1.3	Japanese Clear Soup, 4.2.6	Seafood Stew, 4.2.18
FRI	Lemon Ginger Detox Tea, 4.1.10	Oxtail Soup, 4.2.13	Seafood Broth, 4.2.17
SAT	Strawberry Spread w/ toast	Chicken Vegetable Pasta Soup, 5.2.1	Grilled Salmon Steaks, 5.3.1
SUN	Apple Cider Sausage, 5.1.2	Asian Chicken Salad, 5.2.2	Fiesta Chicken Tacos, 5.3.2

WEEK 2 : LOW RESIDUE DIET

The Rebuilding Phase: Once the flare subsides, slowly reintroduce fiber-rich foods like fruits, vegetables, whole grains and legumes to rebuild intestinal health. Stay hydrated and focus on nutrient-dense, anti-inflammatory fare.

DAYS	BREAKFAST	LUNCH	DINNER
MON	Herbed Avocado Egg Salad, 5.1.6	Broth Braised Asparagus Tips, 5.2.6	Zucchini Lasagna, 5.3.8
TUE	Banana Muffins, 5.1.19	Low Fiber Beet Carrot Soup, 5.2.5	Low & Slow Pulled Pork, 5.3.7
WED	Açai Breakfast Bowl, 5.1.20	Bean and Couscous Salad, 5.2.8	Winter Apple Poke Bowl, 5.3.13
THU	Lemon Ginger Turmeric Drink, 5.1.18	Lemon Chicken Rice Soup, 5.2.7	Fiesta Chicken Tacos, 5.3.2
FRI	Vegetable Frittata, 5.1.13	Greek Yogurt Fettuccini Alfredo, 5.2.11	Tex-Mex Chili, 5.3.11
SAT	Cherry-Mocha Smoothie, 6.1.1	Satisfying Salad, 6.2.2	Curried Quinoa Wraps, 6.3.2
SUN	Pumpkin Overnight Oats, 6.1.2	Cauliflower & Oat Soup with Turmeric, 6.2.4	Pea & Spinach Carbonara, 6.3.6

WEEK 3 : PHASE THREE

The Maintenance Phase: Adopt an overall high-fiber, plant-based diet to promote healthy digestion long-term. Include prebiotics, probiotics, and gut-healing nutrients. Identify personal trigger foods to avoid future flare-ups.

DAYS	BREAKFAST	LUNCH	DINNER
MON	Banana Buckwheat Pancakes, 6.1.23	Satisfying Salad, 6.2.2	Turkey Tortilla Wrap, 6.3.3
TUE	Apple Flax Breakfast Squares, 6.1.25	Roasted Chicken & Winter Squash Salad, 6.2.3	Beef and Lentil Stew, 6.2.3
WED	Peanut Butter & Chia Jam, 6.1.15	Honey Mustard Salmon, 6.2.10	Bean & Spinach Enchiladas, 6.3.9
THU	Breakfast Salad, 6.1.8	Lamb Dhal Makhani, 6.2.11	Beef & Bean Sloppy Joes, 6.3.11
FRI	Coconut-Green Apple Muesli, 6.1.16	Mediterranean Chicken Noodle Soup, 6.2.6	Mexican Quinoa Wraps, 6.3.14
SAT	Sweet Potato Waffles, 6.1.5	High Fiber Pasta, 6.2.8	Bean & Meat Loaf, 6.3.19
SUN	Banana-Nut Oatmeal Cups, 6.1.7	Classic Sesame Noodles, 6.2.12	Grilled Chicken Wrap, 6.3.15

WEEK 4 : PHASE THREE

DAYS	BREAKFAST	LUNCH	DINNER
MON	Freezer Breakfast Burritos, 6.1.17	Salmon-Stuffed Avocados, 6.2.9	Chorizo & Pinto Bean Chili, 6.3.4
TUE	Apple-Oat Energy Balls, 6.1.20	Slow Cooker Black Bean Soup, 6.2.13	Teriyaki Tofu Rice Bowl, 6.3.16
WED	Blue Corn Waffles, 6.1.24	High Fiber Pasta, 6.2.8	Bean & Meat Loaf, 6.3.19
THU	Mocha ProteinOvernight Oats, 6.1.29	Creamy White Bean and Spinach Soup, 6.2.18	Falafel Tabbouleh Bowls, 6.3.27
FRI	Apple-Oat Energy Balls, 6.1.20	Slow Cooker Black Bean Soup, 6.2.13	Teriyaki Tofu Rice Bowl, 6.13.16
SAT	Banana-Nut Oatmeal Cups, 6.1.7	Classic Sesame Noodles, 6.2.12	Grilled Chicken Wrap, 6.3.15
SUN	Pumpkin Overnight Oats, 6.1.2	Cauliflower & Oat Soup with Turmeric, 6.2.4	Fiesta Chicken Tacos, 5.3.2

WEEK 5 : MEAL PLAN

Transition to a high-fiber lifestyle. Aim for 25-30g fiber daily from a variety of plant-based sources like vegetables, fruits, whole grains, nuts, seeds and legumes.

DAYS	BREAKFAST	LUNCH	DINNER
MON	Apple-Oat Energy Balls, 6.1.20	Mexican Quinoa Wraps, 6.3.14	Lentil Fritters, 6.3.1
TUE	Pumpkin Overnight Oats, 6.1.2	Posh Beans On Toast, 6.2.28	Curried Quinoa Wraps, 6.3.2
WED	Blue Corn Waffles, 6.1.24	Turkey Tortilla Wrap, 6.3.3	Chorizo & Pinto Bean Chili, 6.3.4
THU	Bean & Spinach Enchiladas, 6.3.9	Vegetable Frittata, 5.1.13	Beef and Lentil Stew, 6.3.5
FRI	Freezer Breakfast Burritos, 6.1.17	Teriyaki Tofu Rice Bowls, 6.13.16	Pea & Spinach Carbonara, 6.3.6
SAT	Coconut-Green Apple Muesli, 6.1.16	Salmon with Spinach Rice, 6.3.17	Pork Sausage & Green Lentil Braise, 6.3.7
SUN	Banana-Nut Oatmeal Cups, 6.1.7	Bean Chili, 6.3.13	Grilled Chicken Wrap, 6.3.15

WEEK 6 : MEAL PLAN

Emphasize anti-inflammatory foods rich in omega-3s like fatty fish, walnuts, flaxseeds and olive oil. Stay hydrated and limit potential irritants like caffeine and alcohol.

DAYS	BREAKFAST	LUNCH	DINNER
MON	Apple-Oat Energy Balls, 6.1.20	Mexican Quinoa Wraps, 6.3.14	Turkey Tortilla Wrap, 6.3.3
TUE	Mocha ProteinOvernight Oats, 6.1.29	Vegetable Frittata, 5.1.13	Teriyaki Tofu Rice Bowl, 6.3.16
WED	Blue Corn Waffles, 6.1.24	Honey Mustard Salmon, 6.2.10	Mexican Quinoa Wraps, 6.3.14
THU	Breakfast Salad, 6.1.8	Roasted Chicken & Winter Squash Salad, 6.2.3	Falafel Tabbouleh Bowls, 6.3.27
FRI	Peanut Butter & Chia Jam, 6.1.15	High Fiber Pasta, 6.2.8	Grilled Chicken Wrap, 6.3.15
SAT	Coconut-Green Apple Muesli, 6.1.16	Classic Sesame Noodles, 6.2.12	Grilled Chicken Wrap, 6.3.15
SUN	Banana-Nut Oatmeal Cups, 6.1.7	Salmon-Stuffed Avocados, 6.2.9	Pea & Spinach Carbonara, 6.3.6

WEEK 7 : MEAL PLAN

Continue customized high-fiber, anti-inflammatory eating patterns long-term. Focus on gut-friendly fermented foods. Enjoy an occasional "free" meal while being mindful of portions.

DAYS	BREAKFAST	LUNCH	DINNER
MON	Freezer Breakfast Burritos, 6.1.17	Salmon-Stuffed Avocados, 6.2.9	Chorizo Chili, 6.3.4
TUE	Breakfast Salad, 6.1.8	Lamb Dhal Makhani, 6.2.11	Beef & Bean Sloppy, 6.3.11
WED	Banana-Nut Oatmeal Cups, 6.1.7	Classic Sesame Noodles, 6.2.12	Grilled Chicken Wrap, 6.3.15
THU	Bean & Spinach Enchiladas, 6.3.9	Salmon with Spinach Rice, 6.3.17	Beef and Lentil Stew, 6.3.5
FRI	Coconut-Green Apple Muesli, 6.1.16	High Fiber Pasta, 6.2.8	Falafel Tabbouleh Bowls, 6.3.27
SAT	Coconut-Green Apple Muesli, 6.1.16	Salmon with Spinach Rice, 6.3.17	Grilled Chicken Wrap, 6.3.15
SUN	Peanut Butter & Chia Jam, 6.1.15	Classic Sesame Noodles, 6.2.12	Pea & Spinach Carbonara, 6.3.6

WEEK 8 : MEAL PLAN

DAYS	BREAKFAST	LUNCH	DINNER
MON	Herbed Avocado Egg Salad, 5.1.6	Lemon Chicken Rice Soup, 5.2.7	Chorizo Chili, 6.3.4
TUE	Peanut Butter & Chia Jam, 6.1.15	Lamb Dhal Makhani, 6.2.11	Classic Sesame Noodles, 6.2.12
WED	Blue Corn Waffles, 6.1.24	Honey Mustard Salmon, 6.2.10	Bean & Meat Loaf, 6.3.19
THU	Bean & Spinach Enchiladas, 6.3.9	Mediterranean Chicken Noodle Soup, 6.2.6	Falafel Tabbouleh Bowls, 6.3.27
FRI	Apple-Oat Energy Balls, 6.1.20	Slow Cooker Black Bean Soup, 6.2.13	Southwest Chicken, 6.3.20
SAT	Pumpkin Overnight Oats, 6.1.2	Honey Mustard Salmon, 6.2.10	Grilled Chicken Wrap, 6.3.15
SUN	Banana Muffins, 5.1.19	Turkey Tortilla Wrap, 6.3.3	Lentils Fritters, 6.3.1

SUPPLEMENTARY CONTENTS

Unlock Exclusive Culinary Insights!

Scan the QR code below to access four exclusive culinary bonuses included with the "Diverticulitis Cookbook." These resources are tailored to support your journey toward healthier eating and mindful cooking. Embrace these tools to elevate your culinary experience and maintain a flare-up-free lifestyle. Dive into this enriching adventure and continue to uncover delicious possibilities with each page of this cookbook.

If you encounter any issues or have feedback to share, do not hesitate to reach out directly at info@amazing-editions.com. Your input is invaluable as we strive to provide the best possible support to our fellow cooks on the path to a healthier and more fulfilling life. Let the culinary revelations begin!

Conclusion

You will have a thorough grasp of diverticulitis after reading this book. Diverticular illness may be prevented, and its effects reduced by having regular bowel function and preventing constipation. The severity of your problem will determine your doctor's therapy for diverticulitis.

Diverticulitis that is not difficult may usually be managed at home. It's possible that your doctor may advise you to make dietary modifications. They may recommend drugs, such as antibiotics, in certain circumstances. If you have issues due to diverticulitis, you may have to go to a hospital for medical care. An intravenous (IV) line may be used to provide liquids and antibiotics. You may require surgery or another technique depending on the sort of issue. To do so, follow these steps:

Eat more fiber: Fiber draws more water into the stool, making it fuller, softer, and simpler to travel through the colon – and move faster.

 Drink lots of water: Because eating more fiber takes more water, you'll have to drink more water to keep your stool soft and moving. Many doctors recommend that you drink half the body weight in oz.

Exercise daily: Physical activity aids in getting food through the intestines if you can walk for half an hour on most days.

Made in the USA
Las Vegas, NV
03 May 2024

89489981R00057